Intellectual Disability and Being Human

Intellectual disability is often overlooked within mainstream disability studies, and theories developed about disability and physical impairment may not always be appropriate when thinking about intellectual (or learning) disability.

This pioneering book, in considering intellectually disabled people's lives, sets out a care ethics model of disability that outlines the *emotional caring sphere*, where love and care are psycho-socially questioned, the *practical caring sphere*, where day-to-day care is carried out, and the *socio-political caring sphere*, where social intolerance and aversion to difficult differences are played out. It does so by discussing issue-based everyday life, such as family, relationships, media representations and education, in an evocative and creative manner. This book draws from an understanding of how intellectual disability is represented in all forms of media, a feminist ethics of care, and capabilities, as well as other theories, to provide a critique and alternative to the social model of disability as well as to illuminate care-less spaces that inhabit all the caring spheres. The first two chapters of the book provide an overview of intellectual disability and the debates surrounding disability, and outline the model. Having begun to develop an innovative theoretical framework for understanding intellectual disability and being human, the book then moves onto empirical and narrative driven issue-based chapters. The following chapters build on the emergent framework and discuss the application of particular theories in three different substantive areas: education, mothering and sexual politics. The concluding remarks draw together the common themes across the applied chapters and link them to the overarching theoretical framework.

An important read for all those studying and researching intellectual or learning disability, this book will be an essential resource in sociology, philosophy, criminology (law), social work, education and nursing in particular.

Chrissie Rogers joined Aston University as a sociologist in the School of Languages and Social Sciences in September 2012. She graduated from Essex with her PhD (ESRC) in Sociology (2004) and then secured an ESRC post-doctoral fellowship (Cambridge). She subsequently published a monograph, *Parenting and Inclusive Education*. Chrissie has held posts at Keele, Brunel and Anglia Ruskin. She has published in the areas of mothering, disability, intimacy, and sociology of education, and also completed a small piece of research with young disabled people on relationships, friendships and leisure time. Chrissie co-edited *Critical Approaches to Care* with Dr Susie Weller and is editing a special issue for *Sexualities* on intellectual disability and sexuality. Chrissie is also writing in the area of women in the academy, and co-construction of research with disabled people.

Routledge Advances in Disability Studies

New titles

Towards a Contextual Psychology of Disablism
Brian Watermeyer

Disability, Hate Crime and Violence
Edited by Alan Roulstone and Hannah Mason-Bish

Branding and Designing Disability
Reconceptualising Disability Studies
Elizabeth DePoy and Stephen Gilson

Crises, Conflict and Disability
Ensuring Equality
Edited by David Mitchell and Valerie Karr

Disability, Spaces and Places of Policy Exclusion
Edited by Karen Soldatic, Hannah Morgan and Alan Roulstone

Changing Social Attitudes Toward Disability
Perspectives from historical, cultural, and educational studies
Edited by David Bolt

Disability, Avoidance and the Academy
Challenging Resistance
Edited by David Bolt and Claire Penketh

Autism in a De-centered World
Alice Wexler

Disabled Childhoods
Monitoring Differences and Emerging Identities
Janice McLaughlin, Edmund Coleman-Fountain and Emma Clavering

Intellectual Disability and Being Human
A Care Ethics Model
Chrissie Rogers

Intellectual Disability and Being Human

A care ethics model

Chrissie Rogers

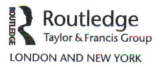

LONDON AND NEW YORK

First published 2016 by Routledge

2 Park Square, Milton Park, Abingdon, Oxon OX14 4RN
711 Third Avenue, New York, NY 10017, USA

Routledge is an imprint of the Taylor & Francis Group, an informa business

First issued in paperback 2017

British Library Cataloguing in Publication Data
A catalogue record for this book is available from the British Library

Library of Congress Cataloging in Publication Data
Rogers, Chrissie, author.
Intellectual disability and being human : a care ethics model / Chrissie Rogers.
p. ; cm. -- (Routledge advances in disability studies)
Includes bibliographical references and index.
ISBN 978-0-415-66458-5 (hbk) -- ISBN 978-1-315-63871-3 (ebk)
I. Title. II. Series: Routledge advances in disability studies.
[DNLM: 1. Intellectual Disability. 2. Mentally Disabled Persons--psychology. 3. Personhood. 4. Standard of Care--ethics. WM 300]
RA790.5
362.2--dc23
2015034993

ISBN: 978-0-415-66458-5 (hbk)
ISBN: 978-1-138-10323-8 (pbk)

Typeset in Times New Roman
by Taylor & Francis Books

For Sherrie – always

'Why does society have so little time, space and care for intellectually disabled people? This is the vital question Chrissie Rogers takes on here to offer both a challenge to our care-less society and an alternative imaginary for how we could live care-fully. Through a strikingly innovative account that draws on philosophical ideas, empirical research and cultural analysis, this book makes a powerful and emotive case for a care-ethics model of disability that fills important gaps in existing approaches to critically thinking about intellectual disability.'

— *Professor Janice McLaughlin, Professor of Sociology,*
Newcastle University, UK

Contents

Acknowledgement

Acknowledgements are a strange thing to write, as they can feel a little like an Oscar winning list of thank yous. Nevertheless a book does not get written in a vacuum – as such. Although it might feel like it. Much of the time a book has taken months, if not years to write, with lecturing and administration and other such stuff to punctuate the writing and thwart the muse. If you're lucky, that is all that makes for failing to meet yet another deadline. However, in many cases, mine included, life has hindered, if not at times immobilised my writing in quite significant ways. Namely, my health issues, with endoscopies, Barret's diagnosis, and serious chest infections that lasted a whole summer, along with a broken wrist and total abdominal hysterectomy only months ago, all having an impact. Then there was my daughter's ill health, when I wondered if we were actually going to see every consultant, but with MRIs she was diagnosed with Chiari malformation, on top of her already disabled M-CM identity. It was, and still is a worrying time. Fortunately my husband has remained consistently healthy. Although his time as head of department during this book writing process was not a walk in the park. Yet, it is finished, and for that I can only thank my daughter, Sherrie Tuckwell, who always sees me at my desk, just down from her bedroom, and my husband Eamonn Carrabine, who pretty much gave up some of his sabbatical to 'care for' me during my post-operative phase. The significant people in my life have always been there. Yet I have to also thank Eamonn as a peer too. He picked up my manuscript when I cried, saying 'I can't do this', and skimmed it, telling me off for idiosyncratic stylistic foibles. He put in a comment box 'Eugh' when I wrote 'unpack' and chastised me for writing 'interestingly' too much. I think these things have been ironed out!

I have indeed been lucky enough to gain support from my department (Sociology) at Aston University, as this final push has been during a sabbatical. I am truly grateful for that. I am also fortunate to have brilliant colleagues, but Sarah Jane Page and Katy Pilcher have managed to take me away from work for cocktails every now and again. That of course was always useful and necessary. I would like to note with thanks some academics – known and not known to me personally – who have influenced my work in a significant way. Eva Kittay, Kathleen Lynch, Martha Nussbaum, John Vorhaus, Ken

Plummer, Ian Craib, Jonathan Herring, Tom Shakespeare, Mike Oliver, and many feminist care ethics scholars. There are other scholars, clearly, but all of these have made me think more deeply about the world we live in and disability more specifically. In addition, Katherine Runswick-Cole and Dan Goodley consistently made me aware of what was going on with LB, as while I just wrote about intellectual disability they were out there doing stuff! And of course on that note, I thank Sara Ryan and LB for being such an influence on this book and my life. I would like to thank Tam Sanger for a big proof read on an almost finished draft. If I didn't do something though, it's all my fault. Finally all my family are brilliant and are always a support, especially Mum, Dad and sisters, and all the people in this book from interviews gathered will remain influential and inspirational.

A note on the text

There are scattered throughout references to and excerpts from my previous work, all of which are in the bibliography. That said, much of the narrative is new and wholly original, and the setting up of the care ethics model has not been written about by me, elsewhere, as yet.

1 Introduction

Being human

Introduction

> Imagine a society in which the generation of wealth is the primary goal. Where success is measured solely by income. Children are left uncared for by parents obsessed with generating more income. Older people are left in squalid conditions, provided with the minimum level of care by the lowest paid workers. Those who could not face leaving their parents or children in these dire situations and undertook care themselves are left in poverty and social exclusion. Exhaustion, loneliness and hardship are the order of the day for these carers, even if cheered by the rewards of the caring itself. Women who undertake the majority of care and make up the larger portion of older people suffer significantly more than men. The ever increasing number of older people is seen as a nightmare scenario, a route to catastrophe, rather than a cause to celebration. Disabled people are viewed as a burden and inconvenience.
>
> (Herring, 2013: 320)

When I read *Caring and the Law* by Jonathan Herring (2013) this quote stood out and captured much of what I had been considering while writing. I look at his work in a little more detail in Chapter 2, but for now, I simply want to use this evocative, yet meaningful way of imagining society and ask these questions, specifically in regards to intellectual disability. Namely because my research answers these questions with yes, and this is unacceptable. So I ask, can you imagine a society where a child is excluded from any meaningful education because of their intellectual impairments, or a mother who is troubled with suicidal and murderous thoughts because she feels alone in her community? Can you imagine a society where a young woman is sexually assaulted by her school peers, and no one believes her, or a society where meeting a friend is always a struggle and having a baby is inconceivable? Can you imagine a society where a young man dies in a bath, in care? Just imagine a society where an intellectually disabled adult is poor, excluded, shamed and left without dignity or respect (see also Vorhaus, 2016). Thinking through these questions and issues, this book draws upon empirical research, personal reflections and theoretical discussion in an attempt to provoke responses and action for a deeper understanding and change-making process regarding the private troubles and public issues (Wright Mills, 1959) that permeate intellectual disability.

Intellectually disabled people have generally been excluded and previously there has been no political movement to do anything about this (Carlson, 2005, 2010; Carlson and Kittay, 2010). This book therefore is premised on proposing a care ethics model of disability, so that we can begin to map, understand and take forward caring and care-full work, not only for intellectually disabled people but for *all people*. I suggest there are three spheres of caring and care-full work, but these are currently populated with many care-less spaces.

- *The emotional caring sphere*

  where love and care are psycho-socially questioned

- *The practical caring sphere*

  where day-to-day care is carried out relationally

- *The socio-political caring sphere*

  where social intolerance and aversion to difficult differences are played out.

These three spheres interact in complex ways. They are the foundation of a care ethics model of disability and are grounded in social and political relations that seek caring legal and cultural processes. Ultimately I suggest a need to contemplate caring work and relationships rather than care work *per se*.

Thinking about and imagining care, social justice, ethics and social inclusion in the context of intellectual disability is tricky, especially when, by comparison to physical disability, far less has been written about intellectually disabled people's lives, and particularly about those with profound and multiple impairments (Vorhaus, 2016). As a heterogeneous group they are not considered full citizens, they certainly struggle to be heard, and at worst are dehumanised (Carlson, 2010). Also there is often talk of giving people a voice, but I am not suggesting here that we give people a voice as such; they already have one – whether that is verbal or otherwise. Yet I do not want to lose sight of the fact that those who 'speak', or are 'speaking with', or being 'spoken for' are not being listened to. Moreover, a challenge arises when those in power make decisions based on attributes such as rationality, language, and roughly equal physical and mental capacity, as rudiments for participating in citizenship (Nussbaum, 2006). *This clearly excludes many intellectually disabled people from contributing to, and participating in, civil society.* However, participation in social, and one might argue political, life is essential to being human, in whatever form that might take. After all, Hannah Arendt (1998: 7) reminds us that the language utilised by the Romans, who were perhaps the most political of people, used the words 'to live' and 'to be among men' or 'to die' and 'to cease to be among men' [*sic*]. Therefore, '[n]o human life, not even the life of a hermit in nature's wilderness, is possible without a world which directly or indirectly testifies to the presence of other human beings' (Arendt, 1998: 22).

Human beings live together, regardless of their intellectual capacity, relationally and with reciprocity (Vorhaus, 2016). Their labour (life itself), their work (worldliness), and their action (serving political bodies) make up the human condition of being together (Arendt, 1998). Notably the Maasai people in Kenya believe that the definition of being human is to live among people, and other cultures define being a person in relation to kinship ties rather than individual ability (Stienstra and Ashcroft, 2010). I am not criticising Western capitalist society here through comparison to other cultures or suggesting for one moment that inhumane atrocities do not occur across the globe. Also I do not propose that being alone is inhumane or dehumanising. Nevertheless, carelessness, exclusion, lack of love and friendships, oppression and incarceration *are* dehumanising. As, '[p]eople do not spring up from the soil like mushrooms. People produce people. People need to be cared for and nurtured throughout their lives by other people, at some times more urgently and more completely than at other times' (Kittay, 2005: 1; see also Geertz, 1973). Thus, the *emotional caring sphere,* where love and care are psycho-socially questioned, the *practical caring sphere,* where day-to-day care is carried out and the *socio-political caring sphere*, where social intolerance and aversion to difficult differences are played out are critical when considering intellectual disability. This is largely because particular discourses around genetic disorders, normative social interaction, and reflections on what it means to be human seem to suggest that intellectually disabled people are better off dead or denied existence (Habermas, 2003; Pfeiffer, 2006; Shakespeare, 2006; Slee, 2011, 2012; Stienstra and Ashcroft, 2010). I suggest, however, that this is not the case. Political life, education and citizenship, family and care-full practices, representations of disability, personal and intimate relationships, and other such aspects of social life ought to be at the forefront of social and political change; not pity and tolerance at best, abuse and murder at worst.

Indeed, throughout time intellectually disabled people have caused more than a little concern for the legal system, policy makers, social cohesion and reproduction, and the vitriol that has been levied at them, and about them, in the past century is evident. As David Pfeiffer quotes from past social reformers and eugenics protagonists, 'feebleminded' people are '"an evil that is unmitigated", a poison to the race, and their "very existence is itself an impediment" to civilization' (2006: 83). Intellectually disabled people have been abused, stigmatised, excluded, violated, controlled and killed, and yet they are human beings embodying personhood. A century or more of violence, implicit or explicit, towards particular people needs radical reform, politically, legally, socially and psycho-socially, because if other humans, those in power, those in everyday life, agree that intellectually disabled people are beneath them on some kind of human hierarchy, then the task is hopeless. I do not adhere to the notion that the task is hopeless, but see it as a struggle nevertheless. Indeed, we still have some way to go, as Eva Kittay (2010) suggests, with certain realms of philosophy remaining fixed on the notion that intellectually disabled people can be likened to pigs and dogs when it comes to being human and non-human.

This was highlighted in an open discussion at a conference, where Kittay was asked by the presenter, a fellow philosopher, 'well, can you tell us some of these morally significant psychological capacities in which you think that human beings, and let's talk about real ones, so the ones who are "profoundly mentally retarded", to use that term, in which they *are* superior to [...] pigs or dogs' (Kittay, 2010: 408 [emphasis in original]) and as Kittay shakes her head at this question, the speaker says 'you have to put up or stop saying that' (2010: 408). Kittay believes that intellectually disabled people are superior to dogs and pigs. Essentially the speaker wanted to hear Kittay's view on the psychological differences (regarding capacity) between these animals and intellectually disabled people and if she could not do that, she was to keep her mouth shut; she was to remain silent. Anecdotal this might be, but we are talking about academics who teach future philosophers and promote the moral acceptability of killing impaired foetuses – enabling emotional distance for the student. This is preferable, for some philosophers, to discussing with students real intellectually disabled adults living everyday human lives, and then contemplating their rights to life (Kittay, 2010). Therefore, considering science, eugenics and norms regarding human life, Lennard Davis, for example, suggests a link between eugenics and statistics that is largely due to the fact that the 'central insight of statistics is the idea that a population can be normed' (2006: 6)[1], meaning we can have standard and non-standard populations ('normal' and 'abnormal') and therefore standard and non-standard human beings. Reflecting upon the 'standard' and 'non-standard' human being can be particularly useful in times when there is confusion and uncertainty around scientific research such as bioethics and the 'right to life', spurious links between autism and immunisations, the rhetoric of 'inclusive' education for disabled children, oppressive disablism and sexism, representations of disability as well as difficult experiences for family members or others caring for and with disabled children/adults.

Normalcy: the politics of sameness and being human

The hegemony of normalcy is, like other hegemonic practices, so effective because of its invisibility. Normalcy is the degree zero of modern existence. Only when the veil is torn from the bland face of the average, only when the hidden political and social injuries are revealed behind the mask of benevolence, only when the hazardous environment designed to be the comfort zone of the normal is shown with all its pitfalls and traps that create disability – only then will we begin to face and feel each other in all the rich variety and difference of our bodies, our minds, and our outlooks.

(Davis, 1995: 170–171)

Normalcy is pervasive as we 'live in a world of norms' (Davis, 2006: 3).[2] Moreover, these norms relate to the human, personhood, civilisation, morality, the body, health and so on. But is there any point in discussing norms and normalcy, when, quite obviously, to be 'normal' is not necessarily something that you are or that is; and really, who wants to be this 'normal'? Normality is a perception rather than a reality, yet more often than not differences are positioned as 'malformed', 'defective', spoilt, stigmatised, or 'deformed' (Davis, 1995; Goffman, 1990). However, that is not to say that to *feel* any of these differences is not an experienced reality and damaging or dangerous to the human being. By reflecting upon history in relation to difference, with respect to both aesthetics and intellectual capacity, I understand that recent past narratives form discourses on tolerance and have been woven into legislation and cultural perceptions of 'abnormality'. After all, to 'tolerate' something or someone is more appealing than persecution or prejudice, and the latter has been obvious to many on the receiving end of this. Yet, when a person is tolerated for their behaviour or what they look like, they are put up with, not necessarily accepted; this could be considered violent. I suggest that difference (and diversity) ought to be embraced rather than negotiated in yet another attempt to normalise the human being. Indeed tolerance, ideologically, is the dark side of diversity as neoliberalism utters empty rhetoric (see also Davis, 2013). We need to recognise that we are all distinctive; to look away and deny difference is inhumane and care-less.

Hence, to be aesthetically normal, to behave within a set of social norms, may be both culturally and historically specific, but has social change via modernity described and prescribed what 'normal' is in an attempt to create a more desirable being, based on that which is undesirable? In the case of disability and impairment, a girl who dribbles so much that she wears a rolled up hanky in her mouth; a boy who bangs his head with his hand when distressed; a teenager who is unable to construct a sentence on paper and a child who is unable to negotiate sexual/social boundaries are all considered 'abnormal' and deemed to 'lack something' – the regular human condition? They do not fit into the construction of what it is to act in a socially acceptable way – to be a fully functioning human being. Who defines this norm? Who says what is normal and what is not? The socio-political caring sphere, including the 'experts', social media, image makers and politicians, all seem to play a part in the dissemination of knowledge around differences and sameness, but how is this constructed? What is a 'normal' image, behaviour, education, pupil, mother, family, friend or lover? For example, in the case of intellectual disability and education, the identification and assessment of a learning difficulty in the UK is a process tied up in a language that privileges good behaviour and academic attainment. In thinking about this construction of a norm, does 'normal' behaviour, intellect, aesthetic presentation, mothering, friendship and intimacy make us human – no it does not.

Philosophically, on being human, Frierson (2013) asks, what can I know, what ought I to do, what may I hope, and ultimately, what is the human being? He does so by interrogating Kant's work in detail. Of course, simply put this could be problematic in the case of intellectual disability for not all people have the capacity that enables self-reflection and agency as we know it (Vorhaus, 2016). Actually asking the question, as I do here, 'what is a human being?' (or rather 'what is it to be human?') really means thinking about 'who am I in relation?' If a human being is fractured, intellectually, aesthetically, physically, emotionally, then the vulnerability of a sense of self, our own being, is questioned, even if that is reflected upon with someone else. What Frierson (2013), through Kant's anthropologies, attempts to do is to understand the human being. Crudely put, the three anthropologies of Kant's that Frierson (2013: 6) uses are: *transcendental* (how one should think, feel, choose), *empirical* ('scientific' observation-based descriptions and how the human being might feel, think, act), and *pragmatic* (pulling together the transcendental and empirical). This is largely all considered in relation to a norm. For example, transcendental anthropology 'characterises the process of thinking, judging, choice, and aesthetic appreciation from-within' (Frierson, 2013: 12), and this is important in evaluating a 'normative dimension' (Frierson, 2013: 13). It is this aspect that is of interest in this book, as through the lens of the visual, the intellectual, the relationship and the familial 'norm', we can begin to understand the human being in relation to the three caring spheres: the *emotional*, the *practical*, and the *socio-political*. Critically, however, transcendental anthropology 'focuses on what can be known about human beings *a priori* through an examination of basic mental faculties "*from within*" that specifically attends to the *conditions of possibility* of *normative* constraints on human beings' (Frierson, 2013: 13, emphasis in original). Although interesting, this is hugely problematic for intellectual disability research as 'from within' is not necessarily active or obvious. Further, it is irksome when attempting to consider relationships and care ethics. So rather than thinking from within, I want to move to the other extreme in thinking about being human, and consider how imagining occurs beyond the self, but always in relation. It might be that we make meaning, or make sense of our world and we consume images and interact with storytelling all while we construct care-full and care-less spaces.

Looking away, imaginings and care-less spaces

Disgusting, dangerous, shameful creature

Turning away from normalcy, I understand that people often make assumptions about the lives of others largely based on what they know, or indeed think they know, and this is often as a result of imaginings – the imagination. I began this book by asking the reader to imagine a society so bad, so inhuman; but often it is not easy to imagine others' lives without imagery or a cultural context. As Iris Marion Young suggests, people are often ignorant about others' lives. She argues that 'perhaps more often people come to a situation of political discussion with a stock of empty generalisations, false assumptions, or incomplete and biased pictures of the needs, aspirations and histories of others' (Young, 2000: 74). As such these assumptions about other people are often dependent on a limited focus or stereotype based on representation, creative narratives and everyday images. With regards to disabled people, the story which is often told is that their lives are 'joyless, that they have truncated capabilities to achieve excellence, or have little social and no sex lives' (Young, 2000: 74), are always in need and offer little in the way of economic growth and that they are therefore less than human. Martha Nussbaum speaks to the issues pertinent to humanity, being human and intellectual disability; for example, *Hiding from Humanity* is a thesis on disgust and shame. These discussions are important in our imaginings, not least because the 'very presence of the mentally handicapped [*sic*] and the physically disabled in our communities, functioning in the public eye, has often occasioned disgust; and yet it would be difficult to maintain that they pose a danger to the social fabric' (Nussbaum, 2004: 79). However, this will always depend on the interpretation of danger. This danger might be that of reproducing disability.

To make a point here about reproducing disability, the 'better off dead' narrative is pervasive in popular media storytelling. For example, in the UK, on BBC Radio 2, *The Jeremy Vine Show* (21 August, 2014) involved a live discussion about whether or not disabled adults 'choose' to have children based on the possibility of their child inheriting their disability. The main guest had a form of brittle bone disease and had suffered through many years of operations and disabling pain. If she were to have a child the chances of her child inheriting the condition would be 50/50, and, were she to conceive, her own body would suffer greatly. She and her husband did not want to risk any of this, and so decided against having their own biological children. This guest categorically said that she was not suggesting that disabled people ought not to live, and that everyone in her situation has a 'choice to decide' on whether or not to go ahead and have a baby. The subsequent phone-in predominantly resulted in those who had pondered this 'choice' and decided not to have their own biological children based upon their particular disabling conditions, for example, for fear of passing on Asperger syndrome or coeliac disease. But there was also a mother who rang in and told the audience she was devastated to see her son in pain as he had inherited an aggressive form of Crohn's disease. The discussion led onto a debate about how certain types of disability can be taken out of the equation as genetic manipulation enables the extraction of particular genetic markers after conception, and, as Vine pointed out, this will increase as biotechnology advances. This reproduction narrative via the news media might be couched in avoidance of pain, but the implicit messages are simple, as I have said: that disabled people are better off dead. The narrative often medicalised and based on economics, is discussed, for example, via assisted suicide narratives where killing disabled people is a rational choice (Haller, 2010). This is in opposition to the social model of disability that activists have fought hard for (Oliver, 1990; Oliver and Barnes, 2012), and further, media messages often merge those who are terminally ill with disabled people, despite these two groups frequently not having parallel everyday experiences (Haller, 2010).

My point here is not to discuss eugenics (it is touched upon in Chapter 5), important as that is, but to argue that this broadcast, reaching mainstream lunchtime audiences, while having an open dialogue, did imply that it is more humane or indeed ethical to avoid a disabling condition.[3] How care-less. This is how it felt for me as a listener, but of course we each have our own relationship to the images we see and the stories we interact with. However interpreted, this example is simply one discussion via the media about the worth of particular disabled lives. But these narratives are constantly leaking into everyday life, in all types of representations and imaginings of disability; they flow in and out. In another example, we find a similar narrative in the news media where a British UKIP (United Kingdom Independence Party) member called for compulsory terminations of foetuses with Down syndrome and other such disabilities in his manifesto (Walker and Quinn, 2012). Despite his suspension, and the outcry from some sectors, it remains the case that some people do consider eugenics (or other forms of eradication) to be a way forward for people who are deemed not fully human (see Haller, 2010) and potentially unable to contribute to society, economically at least. Different images and narratives inform ways of seeing, viewing and interacting that are not necessarily ethical, are therefore unjust (Carrabine, 2012; Jones, 2010; Sontag, 1979, 2003), and subsequently feed the psycho-social. Individuals and communities interpret meaning as follows: 'Objects, people, events in the world – do not have in themselves any fixed, final or true meaning. It is us – in society, within human cultures – who make things mean, who signify' (Hall, 2013: 45). Therefore, as we interact with these stories, we imagine, at the very least, our relationship with death, disability, invalid and unviable human lives. We then make a judgement.

Significantly Nussbaum maintains that we are often happy with, or at least marginally tolerant of, sexism and racism, which do in fact have an enormous detrimental impact on the social fabric of society (see also Young, 1990). However, we often avert our gaze from a dribbling disabled person or move away from someone with 'peculiar' bodily movements and cringe at those who shout incoherently at (seemingly) socially inappropriate moments. This is certainly the case in my research, where a mother did not want her autistic son in the same room as a 'head banging' intellectually disabled child (Rogers, 2007a), and in my previous employment as a residential social worker, where people have moved away from me on the underground tube when accompanied by an obviously intellectually disabled adult. It is also evident in Iris Marion Young's (1990) work where she, as mentioned above, talks about how we see different others all the time, but that this seeing, and likening to our own fragility and frailty, our humanness, makes us want to avert our gaze even more (Young, 1990: 146–7). We also see this looking (or moving) away in other areas, such as in denying mass atrocities (Cohen, 2001) and obstructing or remodelling 'inclusive' education (Slee, 2011). Even

Miller (1997: 37), in his thesis on disgust, offers the reader the opportunity to 'look away' via a quote from Chaucer's prologue to the Miller's Tale: 'Turn over the leef and chese another tale', due to the 'disgusting' nature of his work.

Yet we tolerate violence in the street as part of our corrupt society, we 'forget' that millions of women of childbearing age are dying with HIV- and AIDS-related diseases, turn against those refugees who die as they flee danger, and ultimately we accept (or even participate in) sexism and racism on a global scale. But gazing at intellectually (and physically) disabled people via an image, or in our physical presence, is a reminder that we are frail and vulnerable as human beings. This reminder about the vulnerable human being is not new, as Swift's (1967) eighteenth-century character Gulliver displays. For example, in the final book of *Gulliver's Travels,* Gulliver despairs at his likeness to his human kin and despises his wife and children (and himself) because they are part of the disgusting human race of Yahoos. He cannot contemplate being related to these 'creatures' who are ugly, weak, without grace or morals, and who live without reason. Gulliver had been travelling and had stumbled upon a race of Houyhnhnms (intelligent, civilised horse creatures). The horror of realising he was a Yahoo was too much as the Yahoos made no use of reason other than to 'improve and multiply those vices, whereof their brethren in this country had only the share that Nature allotted them. When I happened to behold the reflection of my own form in a lake or a fountain, I turned away my face in horror and detestation of myself' (Swift, 1967: 327).

For many people in the twenty-first century, the idea of being dependent (and recognising that it will come to most of us, if not in our prime) feels scary at best. As I have acknowledged, we also do not want to think about reproducing impairment, as there is, according to Nussbaum's (2004) critical reflection, no meaning to the life of one who cannot contribute to society and production. Looking at one aspect of Miller's (1997) position on disgust, he, along with Nussbaum (2004) (and Swift, 1967), sees contamination as an important aspect of social and human reactions, and notes there is a hierarchical condition here, with people who are 'disgusting' at the bottom of the pile (see also Rogers, 2007a; Shakespeare, 1994). Likewise, we find in Boyne's (2006) novel, *The Boy in the Striped Pyjamas,* his depiction of a different story of horror and inhumanity when it comes to the destruction of a race; in this example, Jews. This creative narrative, written for young adults, is told through the eyes of a nine-year-old boy who has no idea why Jews are considered disgusting, contaminated and locked away behind a fence. The boy had no understanding of the vehement repugnance levied at this race. The innocence is moving as he befriends a Polish boy through the wire enclosure, in a narrative that ends tragically for them both. The importance for us here is that this underlines the *historical meaning, social conditioning* and *imagining* of how we might interact with each other. This is compounded by the pervasive images we consume.

In thinking about disgust as an emotion and then imagining those who are deemed less than human, we are lured into a belief that certain types of people are contaminated, so for example, homosexuals, 'benefit scroungers', refugees, women, dalits (untouchables), obese people, minority ethnic groups, as well as those with physical and intellectual impairments. Moreover, particular groups of people can all then potentially provoke visceral reactions due to their very existence. This is evident throughout different epochs, across different cultures and via different media. As well as within fiction, as I highlight with Swift and Boyne's narratives, imaginings are also conveyed via social media, news media, film, pictures and art works. As Berger (1972) suggests, seeing comes before words, and we look before we speak. Moreover, the way we actually see things is evident here in what we already know, or do not know. For example, aversion to contamination is often associated with bodily fluids; faeces, vomit, snot, semen and dribble (interestingly the fluid associated with *only* the human being is the tear [Nussbaum, 2004: 89]), and these bodily fluids are allied to animals, which might suggest we have a problematic relationship with our own animality and leaky bodies (Shildrick, 1997, 2002). So, is disgust and therefore shame (if we become contaminated) constructed within psycho-social imaginings via the *socio-political caring sphere*, and is this relationship with disgust based on imagining and interaction? For example, children do not seem perturbed by their own faeces, the boy in the striped pyjamas did not know about any form of Jewishness and the 'horror' of what that might entail. Even more problematic for us here in thinking about intellectually disabled people, for many human beings what bothers them is the relationship between an intellectually disabled person and their animality, vomit, faeces and irrationality; they are something to fear. As such, disgust and shame are related and might be useful to discuss. Like disgust, Nussbaum talks about shame and claims that it is ubiquitous and that most of us learn to cover our weaknesses (2004: 173). These so-called weaknesses are ever present in imaginings, images, and representations of disability and disabled people as 'blessed or damned' but never entirely human (Gartner and Joe, 1987: 2) and therefore always shamed. I will come back to this shaming, but for now, what we imagine, what we experience, what we read, what we 'see' via the television, Internet and news media does leak into and out of our lives in a complex way, and these are all part of the emotional, practical and socio-political caring spheres. More often than not they are not care-full and caring spheres: they are care-less.

The global reach of images and narratives

'Much of society is exposed to views of disability almost exclusively through mass media' (Haller, 2010: 57), and seeing, imagining and viewing is omnipresent as large audiences passively make meaning or actively engage with large charitable events such as telethons and festivals or on-screen television productions. This aspect of cultural production and reproduction is evident in how 'reality' is represented (Barnes and Mercer, 2003; Hall, Evans and Nixon 2013; Haller, 2010). Davis (2006: 241) suggests there is a 'hegemony of normalcy' and that disabled people are often omitted from culture, but when they are represented this occurs in a particular and often stigmatised way, largely because of our fears, as discussed above (Barnes and Mercer, 2003). This position is not limited to disability discourse. Through the lens of the Frankfurt School, and inspired by Zizek, Colin Cremin (2012) looks at the social logic of late capitalism in discussing guilt fetishism and the culture of crisis industry (COCI). This is significant because as a result of people exchanging guilt for a product, for example, buying environmentally friendly goods as a way to 'save' the planet, 'adopting' an orphan or tiger to 'do our bit', by sponsoring a community so people can educate themselves or purchasing goods from an 'ethical' provider we can 'consume guilt free' (Cremin, 2012: 55). In a more sinister example Cremin talks about fundraising and throwing parties in the name of human rights: 'Disturbing images and narratives about torture and oppression encourage the subject to work to displace them from its conscience. At a "human rights party", the image of incarceration or torture is held at a safe distance, there for us to dance around and enjoy' (Cremin, 2012: 55). The partygoers can have fun while alleviating guilt, relieving any tension, and, as Cremin evocatively states, the party 'polishes the tortured bodies so that they catch our gaze and command our coins. Torture is the perfect excuse for a party' (2012: 55). Indeed Eamonn Carrabine (2012: 467) suggests in relation to meaning-making, aesthetics and torture or horror, 'human misery should not be reduced to a set of aesthetic concerns, but is fundamentally bound up with the politics of testimony and memory'.

This spectator 'sport' is certainly an image that comes to mind when huge numbers of people pledge money during day-long events in the UK, such as Children in Need and Comic Relief. The telethons show images and tell stories of 'tragedy', 'heroism' and 'desperation', while audiences shed tears at the displayed real life stories of despair.[4] But then, like the dancing and partying, these 'tragic' images are punctuated with comedy acts, entertainment and live music, such that people are relieved of guilt by pledging their money and are entertained at the same time. This relationship between guilt and the gaze is discussed by Carrabine, who writes about 'just images'[5] and says 'amidst this relentless flow of images are those that have a distinctive, intimate energy' (Carrabine, 2012: 463), and 'while apathy, boredom and voyeuristic pleasure might characterize much mediated viewing' (Carrabine, 2012: 466) there are occasionally things that happen which disturb or trouble us so much that we are moved out of our comatose state and motivated to engage in such charitable events and telethons, and via the pledging of money, so that everything can remain (or seem to remain) psycho-socially stable (see also Tester, 2001). When it comes to thinking through social injustice in relation to images and narratives of intellectually disabled people we can see this is bound up with cultural domination, where disabled people have far fewer material opportunities (Barnes and Mercer, 2003; Davis, 2006; Shakespeare, 2006) and are represented as less than human in fiction and documentary television alike.

Moving beyond the telethons, we can see that disability narratives are currently reflected in wide-reaching shows attracting millions of viewers. Two quite different representations of disability can be found in Vince Gilligan's *Breaking Bad*, first shown in the USA in 2008 with the final series aired in 2013, and David Benioff and Daniel Weiss's adaptation of *Game of Thrones,* which is still running, but was first broadcast in 2011 and is based on novels by George R. R. Martin. Both of these television shows have won numerous awards, and with *Breaking Bad* gaining entry into Guinness World Records as the highest rated show of all time and *Game of Thrones* beating *The Sopranos* with viewers of over 18 million per episode, how they tell a story does have global influence. We have also, as viewers, changed in the way we watch drama. For example, I was recently out with friends talking over lunch, in this instance about the show *Game of Thrones*. It dawned on me that how we observe, interpret and become involved in these types of dramas is as much a social activity of shared meaning as with any serial drama (soap), yet on a grander scale. However, one difference is that, with these blockbusting dramas, we might binge on them and view them via downloads or as a box set. Nevertheless the sharing of images and representations has not altered how people relate, interact and interpret the meanings portrayed.

What do these two shows offer us in reflecting upon, compounding perceptions of, or refuting disabling images? In *Breaking Bad*, within the first two episodes of Season One we find ourselves being introduced to Walter, a financially insecure and bored chemistry teacher, his pregnant wife and teenage disabled son. The most exciting thing that has happened to him is that on his 50th birthday his wife gave him a 'hand job'[6] in bed, while she sold an item on eBay with her other hand. As an audience member it feels like this show is in some ways stuck in the 1980s, with the dated fashion, house and storyline. But of course events take hold, Walter is diagnosed with lung cancer and it becomes a racy, drug-fuelled crime drama. The teenage son, Walter Jr., has cerebral palsy; he has slurred speech and walks with crutches. The actor who plays Walter Jr., R. J. Mitte, has a milder form of cerebral palsy.[7] In one interpretation, cynically, Walter Jr. is there to represent just another tragic part of Walter's life. After all, he is, to all intents and purposes, a 'failed' chemist (while his closest college peer went on to gain credibility and financial reward), he is financially unstable, is about to become an 'old' father and on top of that has a disabled teenage son. Thus, in the first instance we see Walter Jr. as another disabling condition in Walter's 'tragic' life. As the show goes on Walter Jr. also plays to the common theme of making the main character 'wake up' to not feeling so oppressed by the cards Walter has been dealt. For example, in one scene where the family, including Walter's brother-in-law and his wife, all sit around to convince him to have the very expensive cancer treatment, Walter Jr. shouts at his father, waving his crutch, saying he is a 'pussy', and 'what if you had given up on me?' He goes on to say 'do you think living with this is easy?' (meaning his disabling condition).

As with many disability narratives the main character, Walter in this instance, is made to reflect upon his 'non-disabled' life and is reminded that, despite the fact that he has incurable cancer, living with an impairment such as cerebral palsy must be all the more tragic. In another scene Walter Jr. is again a vehicle, a moral conscience, to make us as viewers see Walter differently. Walter Jr. is being ridiculed by some boys in a shop and the downtrodden Walter, who in many ways resembles Arthur Miller's Willy in *The Death of a Salesman*, at this point suddenly transforms. He walks out the back door, where the audience and his family think he has yet again walked away from confrontation, but then appears at the front door of the shop, knocks the boy to the floor and challenges him, while the lad's friends look on. They all scuttle off mumbling, while Walter's family look on in amazement. The implicit and explicit messages and images about how disability and impairment are perceived prick the conscience, feed the psycho-social and serve the pitying socially unjust imaginings that flow seamlessly into the caring (or care-less) spheres. In reality, all the characters in *Breaking Bad* have flaws, except perhaps for the disabled teenager, Walter Jr. The show is full of twists and turns, but in many ways is also quite traditional in its exposition of the hero/anti-hero. After all, Walter, 'doing right' by his family on one hand, is still cooking and selling methamphetamine (crystal meth) illegally on the other.

Benioff and Weiss's *Game of Thrones* is adapted from George R. R. Martin's novels, of which the first was called *A Game of Thrones*. Quite different from *Breaking Bad*, *Game of Thrones* is a fantasy drama with a huge number of characters. In many ways the people, as in *Breaking Bad*, are all characteristically flawed, except perhaps for Hodor, an intellectually disabled (Frankenstein's monster-like) man,[8] who says nothing but Hodor (his name), and Bran Stark, a young boy who lost the use of his legs early on in the series. Notably, although many of the characters are multi-dimensional, the disability narratives continue to reflect commonly held assumptions about disabling conditions. For example, Shireen Baratheon, Lord Stannis's daughter who has a facial disfigurement, is locked away but able to read well. Bran Stark does not have the use of his legs, yet is able to gain out-of-body experiences of flying and running. Tyrion Lannister has dwarfism, is blamed for his mother's death at his birth, is considered a fool and loathed by his sister and father, yet is studious and is also known for his quick thinking and wit. Hodor makes up for what he lacks in speech and intellect with his physical strength. Without his characterisation it would be difficult for some of Bran's storylines to be taken forward as he has the strength to physically carry Bran, feeding into a 'no brain but physical strength' narrative. It is here, in this critique, that we are left wondering whether fiction that reaches millions reflects societal views, and, in this instance, as with many shows, it feels like this is the case. So the disabled characters are outcasts, marginalised, ridiculed, in need, heroic, or vehicles for a moral conscience. As Haller (2010: iii) suggests, 'media narratives that ignore, devalue or misrepresent disability issues reflect the ableism of society through those narratives' and media narratives, whatever form they take, are 'shaped by dominant societal beliefs about disability that come from the power of the dominant able-bodied culture, which defines and classifies disability'.

In pondering these representations of disability via charity telethons, 'pity parties' and wide-reaching television shows, the audience, discussed by Carrabine (2012) in his exploration of 'just images', can move out of their mundane, exhausted lives and gain pleasure from an 'intimate energy'. Yet there is still an attempt to distance their self from an infantilised, awkward, dirty and pitiful Other. But Iris Marion Young (1990), in the broader context of justice and politics of difference, talks about 'cultural imperialism' and interestingly sees the Other as *not* vastly different, stating that,

> discursive consciousness asserts that Blacks, women, homosexuals, and disabled people are like me. But at the level of practical consciousness they are affectively marked as different. In this situation, those in the despised groups threaten to cross over the boarder of the subject's identity because discursive consciousness will not name them as completely different.
>
> (Young, 1990: 146)

She goes on to say that because we see these Others 'face to face', or, I would argue, in different forms of media and images, we are driven to turn away with 'disgust and revulsion' (Young, 1990: 146), or we have to reflect upon our own flawed characters, which is something we would rather not do. With such far-reaching media representations, these Others are no longer hidden away. Sociologically we understand that people who are different and 'socially difficult' have been treated with social injustice and a lack of care, and have been made to suffer. The relevance here is in both the analysis of these images and imaginings and in the ways in which people socially interact with these images and then with each other on a daily basis. These imaginings therefore produce a longer term impact on how we might psychically and collectively perceive what it is to be human – or, on the other hand, do we simply ignore and look away?

Shaming violence, horrific violence: turning the other cheek

How we interact comes back to considering reactions to difficult difference, or towards those who are marked in some way. Emotions provoked, such as shame, and to a lesser extent embarrassment, with respect to a human being can be limiting in often inescapable ways. Shame can be a feeling based on a sense of failure to attain particular goals grounded in cultural expectations or on particular stigma that marks you out as uncomfortably different (Goffman, 1990). Shame is largely centred on feelings of inadequacy, a lack of perfection, but also crucially comes about through interaction with others and the self. We can see this played out in *Game of Thrones* via Shireen Baratheon as a young outcast, imprisoned in a tower and away from others due to her facial disfigurement, and with Tyrion Lannister, who experiences shame relating to his dwarfism every day, from the shame of being born (and being told it was his fault his mother died at his birth) to questions about his worth as a 'proper man'. Both experience shame, but as audience members we too become involved in that shaming and are provoked to feel pity and sympathy at best, but from time to time, what we fear, we often stigmatise, reject and sometimes strive to exterminate (Longmore, 1987). Shaming and feeling shamed are amplified through images and discourse such as the television shows, but also within charity telethons, the 'tragic' disabled child narrative and when soap storylines highlight particular 'flaws', and importantly when a storyline in a novel, film or newspaper article identifies a person, family or trait as shameful. For example, not being able to work, being unable to read, being visibly different, or behaving in a socially unacceptable manner.

We can see, imagine and feel this sense of shame when viewing television shows or reading books that highlight difficult or socially awkward behaviour. Shame (and blame) is also experienced by others who are associated with those who are stigmatised, as in Goffman's (1990) 'courtesy stigma'. This is emphasised in various ways, but as a viewer of the 'true story' BBC drama *Magnificent 7*, the life of Maggi (mother of seven children, four of whom are on the autistic spectrum) seems at least partially based on a relationship with shame and embarrassment. Mishaps, apologies and accidents create a large part of the narrative and hence Maggi's life. In one instance, with Christmas upon them, the family are invited to a neighbour's house for a party and Maggi is unsure as to whether to go. They do go and the boys trash the neighbour's bathroom and are socially challenging for other partygoers. The audience enter into this shameful experience and Maggi goes home, shamed by the reaction of others and by her own feelings about being unable to control her children in public. Looking away is not humane and being provoked into feeling shame is dehumanising for the recipient of the shameful experience. This is indeed a care-less space. In whatever light, we tend to see, and consequently imagine, intellectually disabled people as more than human, less than human and therefore different, special, super-human, erotic, otherworldly, monstrous, grotesque, some thing or someone to gaze at in wonderment, avoid in fear, detest with pity.

Feeling embarrassed and shame-full is important in this discussion. Nevertheless there is a more sinister aspect to how an audience, or for the purposes of thinking through care-less spaces and caring spheres, the socio-political (via the psycho-social), might deny, look away or misrepresent intellectually disabled people within news media. Systemic (and physical) violence occurs both implicitly and explicitly. For example, the Glen Ridge gang rape case in New Jersey, USA (Lefkowitz, 1998) highlights how challenging it is for the media to represent the whole story, when the story, the images and the imaginings do not sit comfortably with, or reflect preferred commonly held beliefs. In this case, a 17-year-old intellectually disabled young woman was gang raped with a baseball bat and a stick by a group of 'good guys'. The story did not get represented as one of horror and disgust via the news media. Bernard Lefkowitz, who interviewed over 200 people and examined hundreds of press articles, found that when the boys were arrested, some time after the event, the initial reaction was, '[t]he mayor emphasized that everyone in the town had acted properly. Not only public officials. Just about everybody who lived there had done the right thing and was blameless for what had happened – *if anything really did happen*' (1998: 273, emphasis added). The emphasis on disbelief that this violent act could take place was apparent.

The missing disability narrative is absolutely clear *if* the audience knows it is there, but more often the audience never hear/see the full story in news media representations. Furthermore, sometimes knowing the full story, spectators look away in disbelief and deny or ignore heinous acts. The main response in this case, after the arrests, was one of incredulity, and the telling and re-telling of the account played out, for example as Lefkowitz (1998: 274) says, the 'boys who had everything, nice teenage clothes, nice well-kept houses, and nice respectable, responsible parents [...] you didn't expect gang rapes in Glen Ridge'. I would suggest, if the young woman had been gang raped in an unlit park by a group of youths who were from a disadvantaged/minority back-ground, a vulnerable disability narrative would have been told. But for this young woman, her perpetrators' advantaged backgrounds and her intellectual impairment fracture the story too much. Crucially, she was not always consistent in her own storytelling; she did not always 'act' like a victim, and she was easily manipulated. This intellectually disabled young woman was not really part of the story told, yet she was the lead character, the victim. For those with profound intellectual impairments, images and narratives often misrepresent and damage all areas of life, resulting in a dehumanising process (see also Rogers, in press). With the news media, via social commentary on the BBC and through the press in the USA, relating to very different areas of life – right to life/death and sexual violence – it seems stories and representations do have something to say, but the message is destructive. Intellectually disabled people as *less than human*, are always considered a burden, a drain, in need of care, and ultimately expendable – extinguishable (Kittay, 2010; Nussbaum, 2004; Shakespeare 2006). It is incredible that we look away from 'disgusting images' and horrific stories and find them a space in the psycho-social which Others those who are too different or too distressed. We shame and stigmatise 'freaks', yet we are intrigued by those who are not like 'us'. For example, as we saw above in the representation of a young intellectually disabled woman gang raped in Glen Ridge, she was largely peripheral to the story as told and imagined. It was the well-heeled young male perpetrators who were the focus of the tagline in the telling of this story.

In discussing this aspect of the image and meaning making, John Berger, writing in the 1970s, argues 'image is a sight which has been recreated or reproduced. It is an appearance, or a set of appearances, which has been detached from the place and time in which it first made its appearance [...]

every image embodies a way of seeing' (Berger, 1972: 2). Seeing (and imagining) is often how we make an immediate connection to something or someone, such that images in fiction, news stories, drama, art works, film and social media can shape the way people think and behave. We know that moral panic around certain groups, for example, in the past, mods and rockers, and more recently young men wearing hoodies, Muslim men (Shain, 2011) and refugees, have been considered problematic due to images generated around identity and global events. However, as suggested above, when it comes to narratives and images surrounding intellectual disability we find them bound up in either heroism, such as in the UK's 2012 Olympics 'super-human' narrative, overcoming difficulty, or 'tragic', as television stories unfold in conjunction with charitable events or fictional representations. The uneasiness here is that their existence, those with stigma, their inclusion, will taint, spoil, and contaminate other non-disabled humans. This is compounded by shameful, stigmatising and unjust narratives and images, or pictures and stories that are simply enticing as they take the viewer away from the banality of every-day life. As it is, human beings are 'deeply troubled about being human – about being highly intelligent and resourceful, on the one hand, but weak and vulnerable, helpless against death, on the other' (Nussbaum, 2004: 336). We turn away from this, and in 'the process we develop and teach both shame at human frailty and disgust at the signs of our animality and mortality' (Nussbaum, 2004: 336).

In a similar vein to guilt (for example when giving money to a charity, as with the telethons and pity parties), whether the imagining is via news stories, fiction, drama or other imagery, the audience enter into a relationship with shame. But unlike guilt the audience might *feel* shame sometimes (for not caring enough), whereas the intellectually disabled person *is* shamed, feels shamed and experiences stigma (this does not happen with guilt in the same way). The impact of shame is invidious and can permeate all aspects of social and psychic life. This shame discourse, especially when it comes to intellectual impairment, is today enflamed by the current privileging of educational attainment that, for example, largely depends on scores as a result of examinations that do little more than test memory and occur in the context of inclusive education (Haller, 2010; Slee, 2011). As already evidenced, shame and shaming images can be very dangerous, not just for intellectually disabled people, but for those caring too. Mothers, like Maggi above, often live in shame due to not living up to the expected ideal of what it is to mother (see Rogers, 2007a, 2007b). This aspirational element tied to shame can be very dangerous (Slee, 2011), as I consider later in this book. Therefore we do need to protect dignity against shaming and dehumanisation through the law (Herring, 2013; Nussbaum, 2004). As Nussbaum (2004: 305) says

> no group in society has been so painfully stigmatised as people with physical and mental disabilities. Moreover, many people who would wholeheartedly oppose all stigmatization based on race or sex or sexual

orientation feel that some sort of differential treatment is appropriate for those who are different 'by nature'.

Shaming is perpetuated through the images that we see, imagine, read and feel. Moreover, intellectually disabled people have often been 'denied humanity' and 'the right to live in the world' (Nussbaum, 2004: 306) (see also Haller, 2010; Riley II, 2005). Also, critically, for those mothers who have produced intellectually disabled children, as in the case of children with Down syndrome or other such impairments, stigma is said to be an 'ugly mistake' (Nussbaum, 2004: 306) (see also Desjardins, 2012; Kittay, 2010; Pfeiffer, 2006). Thus, drawing on Goffman's (1990) notion of stigma, some people gain comfort in seeing themselves as 'normal' (Nussbaum, 2004: 218–219), but what is behind this idea of the 'normal' is that the person with the stigma is *dehumanised* and then by virtue of being associated with that dehumanised person the family or one caring are marked with 'courtesy stigma' (Goffman, 1990).

Some liberals might say that there is no room for law and public policy to interfere with emotional well-being, but Herring (2013) would disagree, saying that '[w]e need the law (and more widely) to prioritise caring. Our central focus should be to provide social and legal regimes which promote, enable and protect relationships of care' (2013: 328). But social media and news media, virtual or otherwise, are discriminatory and exclusionary, and any sort of prejudice or marginalisation process has a hugely negative impact upon individuals and groups – these imaginings, and these realities, are why we need a care ethics model of disability. Moreover, the images portrayed via all forms of media impact upon the substantive areas of life discussed in this book, such as education, mothering and intimacy, via all the caring spheres. It is for me to disentangle the care-less spaces that intellectually disabled people and those others involved in their lives inhabit. It is also for me to understand the queering of norms that exist, so the visual, familial, intellectual and friendship norms, all of which find their place in the care-full and care-less spaces. But for the final parts of this chapter I would like to look at the more personal aspect of intellectual disability and then give a short synopsis of the book.

Caring and the personal: political dimension

[P]hilosophical questions that emerge in connection with intellectual disability are matters that not only are worthy of scholarly interest but speak to the deepest problems of exclusion, oppression, and dehumanization; [...] one's proximity to persons with intellectual disabilities should be neither assumed as a basis for participation in this conversation nor grounds for disqualification when speaking philosophically about this topic.

(Carlson, 2010: 3)

This quote is taken from Licia Carlson's work and in response to the often asked question, when people realise she is writing on the topic of intellectual disability: 'Oh do you have a disabled family member?' (Carlson, 2010: 2). The assumption that she would only be interested in this topic if she had a disabled family member began to irritate her. Thus in her work she says, 'I will identify myself as a non-disabled philosopher who, though not entirely personally distant from the issue' believes the matters outlined above, such as exclusion and dehumanisation are worthy of scholarly interest (Carlson, 2010: 2). I can understand this irritation through a different lens.

Although I am the mother of an adult intellectually disabled daughter, I do not myself have an intellectual impairment, such that when reading work written by disabled scholars I feel a little like an outsider and not quite worthy of writing about disability. Furthermore, when I was asked about my research area, especially in the early days of my PhD, it was assumed that I was an 'insider' as a mother (Cooper and Rogers, 2015). So much so that despite the fact I was in the final stages of my funded PhD and on the brink of starting my post-doctoral fellowship, a senior female professor exclaimed, when I announced delight at my funding approval, 'Oh how lovely, I thought you were doing your PhD as a hobby?' I am still bemused and aggravated by her comment 10 years on. As it is Michel Foucault, like countless feminist researchers, said

> Every time I have tried to do a piece of theoretical work it has been on the basis of elements of my own experience: always in connection with processes I saw unfolding around me. It was always because I thought I identified cracks, silent tremors, and dysfunctions in things I saw, institutions I was dealing with, or my relations with others, that I set out to do a piece of work, and each time was partly a fragment of autobiography.
>
> (Foucault and Faubion, 2002: 458)

This quote captures what I sense about much of my 'sociological imagination' (Wright Mills, 1959), so no, my work has never been a hobby, but it does involve the personal. Notably, what Carlson (2010) alludes to above is that there are people who are actually silenced, whether that is because of proximity to those judged as marked, or those who are indeed considered inferior to more powerful others. There are many who are silenced, not just intellectually disabled people. Silencing is a tool of oppression, as 'when you are silenced, whether by explicit force or by persuasion, it is not simply that you do not speak but that you are barred from participation in a conversation which nevertheless involves you' (Ahmed, 2010: xvi). Yet, if we cannot trust powerful others to perform and embody caring, emotionally, practically and socio-politically, can we ever really speak out? As Sara Ahmed argues, '[a] lack of trust can be a reason not to speak' (2010: xvi).

Personal, theoretical or empirical, I would not be writing about intellectual disability in the way I do were it not for the fact that my adult daughter is intellectually disabled. She was born with Macrocephaly-capillary malformation (M-CM), a very rare genetic disorder, and more recently diagnosed with

Chiari malformation, an incurable brain condition. Yet, I do feel strongly about the fact that simply because I experience something, such as disabling conditions, exclusion, prejudice, pity, and so on, it does not mean others are unable to reflect, write and research about private troubles or public issues; something unfamiliar to their own personal experiences. If this were the case, an awful lot of sociological research would not have occurred. When it comes to intellectual disability, I am clear about the fact that I have a personal connection to this area of thought and experience, but of course the empirical research I draw upon is interpreted through a sociological lens. What I reflect upon in doing disability research as a mother, and as a mother with an intellectually disabled daughter doing research, are two different positions on writing about disability and humanity. One position suggests one does not know what it is like to have an impairment, so why write about it; the other is saying research into that which is so familiar may not really be serious sociological research. Both positions bother me as I am aware of both my subjectivity to and distance from intellectual disability and impairment. More than this, I would argue that intellectual disability research and research into that which is human is not parochial and niche, but that the matters discussed here about being human are for all to consider in advocating a *care ethics model of disability*, and that it is for all to ponder and then act.

Personal caring and care-full spaces

In considering caring and care-full spaces it does not take me long to reflect, or take me too far back in time to remember. On 25th February 2015 I went into hospital for a total abdominal hysterectomy. Then in an untimely manner, the week before the planned surgery I broke my wrist walking into work. These two things really made me contemplate my own care needs, in a physical sense but also in terms of the emotional. The human activity that goes on between people ought always to be carried out with caring and care-full-ness. My husband, during those first two months post-op, was more caring and care-full than I could have ever imagined. I was helpless; I could not wash myself with the cast on my arm for six weeks and stitches from hip to hip. Of course I could ask 'who else would do it?' I ask this question with respect to mothering and intellectual disability in Chapter 4. Who else will care when a person is unable to do caring work for themselves? In circumstances such as this, there is privilege in knowing one has a caring other; a mother, daughter, sister, partner, friend, and so on. Yet, that ought not to be the case. I wrote a blog after the hysterectomy, and this was part of an entry not long before I went down to theatre, reflecting upon my surgeon and anaesthetist and the moment I came round post-surgery.

A well dressed, well-groomed ageing man. And on the occasions I've seen him in the past few months always donning a rather dapper tie. Today was no different. He is so calming and kindly and gentle. I've seen a lot of different consultants in the past 6 months with my daughter and myself and not all have his gentle manner. I like him, despite feeling childlike in his presence. Better infantile and slightly helpless, than an angry teen! I sign away my life, or at least my ovaries if anything untoward is discovered in that area when opened up. Otherwise they would survive the internal cull. He touched my hand and looked on like a father. 'You'll be fine, it will all be over soon and no more disruptions to your life', meaning the dreaded heavy periods and so on. In my head I screamed 'give me the heavy period over this – what if I die?! I'm not ready'. The next time I would see him would be just as I'm about to fall into the deepest of sleeps. Goodbye holder of my life, my womb, my past, my future [...] I begin the last trip as myself as it is, down the corridor in my bed. My womb's final journey. I arrive in a small room. Through the doors I see a hustle and bustle of people in the theatre where I am to play the lead. Actually is it me, the surgeon or the anaesthetist who leads this scene?! The anaesthetist arrives by my side all in green – I think? I really really have to work hard not to break down. He says, I vaguely remember, 'hello, how you feeling?' 'Not great, I'm very scared to be honest,' I quiver. I see my consultant who is calming and the anaesthetist puts a cannula in my hand. I have a word with God. He knows, but I remind him I have to look after my daughter so please don't take me yet! The liquid is pushed in the needle on the back of my hand and runs through my veins. I'm away – nothing. No birds or butterflies. [...] Moments later – in my memory time, not real time, I'm back in my hospital room and hubby looks on. Relief in his eyes. Love in his heart. I'm awake! Alive. I made it through the dark unknown journey. On the way I lost my womb, but for now I have my life.

(Rogers, 2015)

Moreover, on coming home to a network of friends too:

Hubby out all day today working. I had friends planned for today! My wonderful friends. So one that I met at uni and shared a house with back in the day turned up with gifts, food and prosecco in hands. Oh she knows me so well (although I did decline breaking open the bubbles just yet!). We had a brilliant few hours catching up, first in the bed chatting. Peppermint tea was made and we continued. But by late morning I felt the need to have a shower! So naked as the day I was born – I stood in front of her. I wonder if we will giggle about this when we are old. I couldn't do much after the cast shower cap was on! I felt incredibly vulnerable, not with this friend *per se*, but just usually if we are naked it is a choice and ... Well it's just different. But we were fine!!

(Rogers, 2015)

As I stood naked in the shower, with my friend or my husband hosing me down, in that moment I was vulnerable. This moment, however, is some other's everyday life (Vorhaus, 2016). For me, in many ways these caring and care-full moments are like bitter sweet gold dust. Beautiful and shiny, yet one moment later, a gentle breeze and they disappear – for me, gladly, as they were surrounded by pain and discomfort. For others they might constitute the everyday-ness of caring or care-less spaces. My point here, in this personal reflection, is that a care ethics model of disability ought to speak to the day-to-day caring. For if it addresses that which is everyday, that which is mundane, in a caring and care-full manner then additional caring costs (emotional and practical) will not seem quite so extraordinary. Caring ought not to be extra-ordinary. Being vulnerable, temporarily or always, ought not to be burdensome or frightening. I 'hear' myself writing this and reflecting, and then pondering, ask, is this not utopian? Quite possibly, but as I deliberate over the care-less spaces to come, I do not feel too bad for wanting to incite change.

Personal caring and care-less spaces

This book has a lot of care-less spaces to discuss, which is why I have felt it necessary that I write about and develop a more care-full, ethical and moral way of doing caring. For me personally, my life is full of care-full and care-less spaces. As said, a mother with a 28-year-old intellectually disabled daughter, and as a teenage lone mother, I indeed have experienced many a caring moment with my mother and others, as well as existed within many care-less spaces I would rather forget. I just want to highlight a more recent care-less moment, within a care-less space that could have ended in a far more tragic way. As it happens, it worked out, to an extent, but institutional and systemic care-lessness was evident and this absolutely leaks into and out of the emotional, practical and socio-political caring spheres in complex ways as is evident here when I wrote about an incident involving the police and my daughter.

> My daughter, a 27-year-old intellectually disabled adult, mildly on the autistic spectrum and who has M-CM, was yesterday morning apprehended at her learning disability club by two police officers. She was arrested, taken in a police car to the station, searched, and relieved of all her belongings and jewellery, finger printed, put in a cell, interviewed, charged and bailed. Luckily, her step father (Professor of Criminology, which they did not know about) was at home, went to the station, and stayed in the cell with her and attended the interview. They said she was caught on CCTV shoplifting in WH Smith (the two times I can corroborate she was actually with me or in bed). This footage was not shown to either my daughter or hubby. TWO big officers! They then called for another (a female). So policing the town and ridding the centre of – who? People like my daughter? She is traumatised, and scared. What concerns me? Yes, my daughter's physical and mental health. But also, is this how it is? What if she were guilty of robbing £18 of stuff over two days (as I say, she

couldn't have been there at the times they say), but is this how the CJS deals with vulnerable adults? It is such easy pickings for arrest figures, but had she not been in the family she is ... maybe in care, or with parents who have difficulties themselves this would likely be processed and she would end up with a criminal record? As it happens I do not know the outcome, in this case, except that Sir Bob Russell has been informed and the IPCC. Hubby and I were thinking about writing on vulnerable young people in the CJS, but we had no idea we would end up at the sharp end. I am flabbergasted that this process even occurred.

(Rogers, 2015)

This particular care-less moment did come to an end, with a letter to the local MP, with us all meeting with the arresting officer, and with an apology, as well as my daughter's newly instated criminal record being wiped. Despite the process ending for my daughter, the haunting impact of her arrest, inhabiting a prison cell for a few hours, the fear of police officers and of venturing alone out of her own house (our home) went on for much longer. Nevertheless, for every case where there is an 'acceptable' outcome, there are other cases where vulnerable young adults, at best, end up with a criminal record, and at worst die in a cell due to a seizure brought on by stress, for example. This particular personal biographical interlude is about the criminal justice system, but within the pages of this book, of the stories told, I recount numerous care-less moments and all within care-less spaces within local government, the health system, the education sector, the community, and broader 'friendship' networks, among others.

I return, therefore, to thinking philosophically about caring and injustice, my position and my responsibility as a mother with an intellectually disabled daughter, and also as a sociologist. Kittay, as a philosopher, also encounters a 'battlefield' where 'claims of political ideals of justice, autonomy, and equality are grounded on a set of competencies or potentials, many of which my daughter most likely does not possess' (Kittay, 2010: 393). She goes on to say that in critiquing her experiences as a mother and philosopher she might expect a terrain

full of land mines, some of which could be anticipated. Others would be discovered only after I had already stepped on them. Unsurprisingly, I have stepped on several, and it has at times prompted me to ask the question: Should I continue? What is to be gained? I want to defend the idea that stopping is a poor choice – for me, for the profession, and for people with cognitive disabilities.

(Kittay, 2010: 393)

All the reasons to continue to speak out about intellectual disability are on the pages to come; these are motive enough to develop a care ethics model of disability.

Synopsis of the book

In the following chapter I explore disability research, feminist ethics of care and human capabilities. In doing so I formulate a care ethics model of disability that frames my understanding of intellectual disability and what it is to be a human. Essentially capitalist society has had an alienating impact upon humanity, yet in mapping a feminist ethics of care, whereby all humans are interdependent and relational, I introduce care-full and care-less spaces. That said, without social justice it can be challenging for this position to be considered as a serious model, particularly within current legal and human rights discourses. However, although a rights position ought to be considered, it is not sufficient in and of itself, as rights for all are not equal when it comes to caring work. Therefore Martha Nussbaum's work is explored and capabilities examined. By considering a feminist ethics of care, capabilities and the law, I find a space where three caring spheres exist – the emotional, practical and socio-political, all of which relate to each other in complex ways and form an analytic tool so as to develop a care ethics model of disability. The subsequent three chapters are cases where I can identify care-less spaces and show how a care ethics model of disability can frame an understanding of education, mothering and intimacy in relation to intellectual disability.

In Chapter 3, I take to task education and identify that over-bureaucratised and over-restricted curriculum is de-humanising and care-less. A lack of creative care-full spaces prevents children and education professionals from reaching their full potential as learners and leaders. The emotional and practical spaces within formal and informal education are stifling, which leaves children in potential danger and teachers looking to leave their chosen career or at the end of their tether and spent in every way. The socio-political sphere further oppresses where rhetoric of inclusion and care masks toxic care-less spaces while attempting to sanitise and fit all children into a particular mould. In this chapter, I turn to Julie Allan via a politics of inclusion and desire, and Martha Nussbaum through the lens of capabilities, so as to understand inclusion, flourishing, desire and shame. Ultimately motivation and creativity are key to a care-full education, not looking away and denial of difficult differences. Chapter 4 builds upon these ideas of shame and denial, but relates more explicitly to care-less spaces for mothers. I take a more narrative approach in identifying care-less and care-full spaces for mothers and those caring for and with intellectually disabled children. As it is, mothering sometimes occurs within extreme conditions and I highlight a case where an avoidable death transpires. Furthermore, it is evident mothers exist in care-less spaces, emotionally, practically and socio-politically, and there are significant caring costs. I identify suffering as a way to understand carelessness and propose that care-full spaces can exist within a suffering context, as suffering is part and parcel of being human. Extreme care-lessness, however, is not. In recognising suffering I also see hope as a care-full space where support can survive. Moreover, it is through the case of Tracy, a mother from my research data, who has two disabled children, that I map morality and humanity in mothering. In the final substantive chapter, I turn to intimacy and friendship as all human beings want to be among people and are relational and interdependent. I identify that making and maintaining friendships is critical in feeling cared for and about, but as it is, geographical boundaries, social and cultural norms and social media have placed a more governed and restrictive element onto intimacy. I find that sex and reproduction does not make us human *per se,* but that being in caring and care-full relationships does. Yet there are restrictions to these relationships that are not always obvious, as I acknowledge from research, personal vignettes and media representations: that is, there is an abundance of care-less spaces. Moreover, there is a profound need to develop caring so as to enable human flourishing. The final chapter makes concluding remarks and simply draws the book to a close.

Notes

1 Davis (2013) more recently turns to discuss diversity, suggesting the end of the normal, as it is more in line with neoliberalist ideology and I would agree in part. Yet in the case of my work, normality as a concept still has mileage in its critique when it comes to intellectual disability.
2 Davis (2006) is referring here to the construction of normalcy where he takes us back to the likes of Quetelet, the French statistician, Defoe's *Robinson Crusoe* and Marx (Davis, 2006: 3–6), in positioning 'the normal' and 'the average'.
3 I cannot argue with avoiding pain and so on, but if we decide which conditions are disabling or not, we begin to categorise impairment within a hierarchy. Then there are those conditions that are not inherited at all. Is it more caring to terminate at birth?
4 For example, on Facebook and other social media sites people narrate their tears at stories told when they are viewing certain shows.
5 With a play on words: just images as in moral and good images, or just images as in simply images.
6 Hand job is a term for someone masturbating another.
7 One might argue that this is a good representation of disability, unlike the non-disabled actor playing a disabled man in *The Theory of Everything*. This film from 2014 was about the life of Stephen Hawking, the well-known theoretical physicist who developed Motor Neuron Disease, a disabling condition. Eddie Redmayne, a non-disabled actor, played Hawking and received critical acclaim for the performance. It could be argued that this part and others such as this ought to be played by disabled actors.
8 Interestingly, although in the novels, Hodor is not a speech impaired adult but is described as a stable boy. Like with Walter Jr., Hodor is a conduit for moral conscience or the psycho-social. It would not work so well if the character were a stable boy.

2 A care ethics model of disability: ways of being human and intellectual disability

Introduction: spheres of caring

In grounding a care ethics model of disability, how we imagine and understand caring practices is critical to mapping intellectual disability and ways of being human, largely because caring 'is not a strange activity which is undertaken by a few brave souls, but it is ingrained into the existence of every person' (Herring, 2013: 45). Moreover, as Mahon and Robinson (2011: 2) suggest, an 'ethics of care that is political and critical must be grounded in the concrete activities of real people in the context of social relations'. In the following chapters I draw upon and interrogate concrete everyday activities that humans experience as mothers, professionals, friends, partners and children, for example. Notably, recognising the human in being human ought to be at the heart of caring and ethics. Even if someone is profoundly intellectually impaired they will have relationships, and those relationships involve caring (Kittay, 2010; Vorhaus, 2016), but not simply in the sense that a person is in need of care for much of their day-to-day life, rather that they are involved in spheres of caring work, emotionally, practically and socio-politically. As a premise for a care ethics model of disability I introduce three spheres of caring work: the *emotional sphere*, where love and care are psycho-socially questioned; the *practical sphere*, where day-to-day care is carried out relationally; and the *socio-political sphere*, where social intolerance and aversion to difficult differences are played out. These three spheres are all related to each other in complex ways. They are the foundation of a care ethics model of disability and grounded in social and political relations that seek caring legal and cultural processes rather than care work *per se*.

The social model: an outdated mode of thought and care-full proposals?

The social model of disability during the 1980s (in the UK) was a groundbreaking way of understanding the differences between disability and impairment, and paved the way for change. Impairment, as defined by the Union of the Physically Impaired Against Segregation (UPIAS), is 'the lack of a limb or part thereof or a defect of a limb, organ or mechanism of the body' (Oliver,

1996: 22). Therefore prior to the social model, the medical model placed emphasis on impairment and, as a consequence, pathologised disabled people. The disability was considered within and the person with impairments in need of repair. As such, disability according to Michael Oliver (1996: 22) was considered 'a form of disadvantage which is imposed on top of one's impairment, that is, the disadvantage or restriction of activity caused by a contemporary social organization that takes little or no account of people with physical impairments'. Therefore, barriers to social and physical inclusion were in place to subjugate those deemed as less than human. Karl Marx has been hugely influential in how we understand oppression, exclusion and suffering (McLellen, 2000; Oliver, 1990, 1996; Oliver and Barnes, 2012) and thus is still important, especially in exploring intellectual disability, at a day-to-day level of experience (emotionally and structurally), as well as philosophically, in how we explore injustice, ethics and being human.

Whilst many writers are increasingly critical of the social model (Shakespeare, 2006; Thomas, 2007), largely because it cannot engage with the actual difficulties brought about by some impairments, it has transported disability into the public and academic sphere, to be understood as a social phenomenon. Importantly, understanding disability through the lens of Comte and Marx, Oliver (1990: 37) saw disabled people as a group oppressed via the 'progressive evolution of reason and humanity'; moreover, institutional 'changes in policy provision for disabled people were determined by changes in the mode of production'. Furthermore, the study of gendered experiences of disability, via Carol Thomas' (1999, 2007) work, has been crucial in understanding women within a materialist feminist framework. However, despite the social significance of disability, Thomas recognises 'impairment effects', which are the everyday and immediate effects of having an impairment: those experiences that are beyond our understanding from a social model perspective. The personal example she gives to highlight this point is that having one hand means that she is never able to pour boiling water from a kettle into a container, with two hands. Her argument is, if the person unable to carry out this two-handed movement is prevented from gainful employment, this would be classified as disablism (Thomas, 2007). As Thomas highlights, this concept of impairment effects has been taken on board and utilised by those who engage with the social model of disability, but she recognises the need for something more regarding particular difficulties in everyday life.

In understanding intellectual disability the social model can seem somewhat alien, as certain difficult behaviours and day-to-day occurrences, whether for the intellectually disabled person or for the one caring, are not eradicated via the processes of a social model of disability. Whilst Thomas' (1999) early work is embedded, to an extent, in the social model, she states that it is not wholly satisfactory as she positions 'impairment effects' as a new form of repression. She suggests that the social model of disability 'poses rather than answers questions' (Thomas, 1999: 26), and that 'disability – like other forms of oppression associated with gender, "race" and so on – is bound up with the level of development of the productive forces, the social relations of production and reproduction, and the socio-cultural and ideological formation which are found in particular societies' (Thomas, 1999: 44). Her main point though, throughout, is that disability is always a gendered experience and that disability studies has much to learn 'from feminist insight on questions of epistemology' (Thomas, 1999: 69). Arguably it is through the writings of the protagonists of the social model (Finkelstein, 1996; Oliver, 1990, 1996; Oliver and Barnes, 2012) that we come to learn a great deal about disability, human production and individual pathology. That is to say, within a social model of disability the focus of human participation and citizenship is on human rights rather than human needs. For example, a physically disabled individual might need to access a building, but cannot gain access due to lack of ramps and so on; yet she has a right (or sometimes a need) to enter spaces in the community. Not to be able to do so is disabling and care-less.

There are continuing discussions about human rights and needs (Dean, 2010), but *needs* do not speak for themselves (Mahon and Robinson, 2011), and often within disability research needs are associated with vulnerability (see Beckett, 2006; Hollomotz, 2011). Both vulnerability and needs have been considered as negative, especially in the context of disability, the social model, care and dependency. This is largely because choice associated with needs is problematic. If, for example, a parent, child, sibling, or partner is incapacitated, in the short- or long-term, as I said in Chapter 1, what 'choice' is there but to care? The law, for example, is abstract. If you give up paid employment to care practically then is that *your choice*? If you take low-paid care work is that *your choice*? Questions ought to be raised in order to challenge this, as 'the imperative to care is such that talk of choice is somewhat fictitious' (Herring, 2013: 83). Indeed, if people 'choose' to care that ought not to lead 'those who undertake heavy care work to be seriously disadvantaged. Why should those who are caring suffer deleterious consequences as a result?' (Herring, 2013: 84). Significantly, Marx (2007) emphasised the importance of human relationships with respect to production, and in his early work related this to the concept of alienation:

> The Alienation of the worker is expressed thus: the more he produces, the less he can consume; the more he creates, the less value he has [...] Labour produces fabulous things for the rich, but misery for the poor. Machines replace labour, and jobs diminish, while other workers turn into machines.
>
> (Marx, 2007: 71).

When I consider what it means to be human, this understanding could mean that unless we produce labour (in this case caring), or goods (caring practices) that are meaningful to us and the community, we lose any sense of being human. We are either a machine, which is inhuman, or cast aside, unable to produce, which is inhumane. Yet I wonder if responsibility (Herring, 2013) and obligation (Korsgaard, 1996, 2009) come into play too in our understanding of being human. These two concepts, responsibility and obligation, conflict with choice, but nevertheless have a part to perform in caring.

Clearly, there are problems with how Marx's theory can be mapped onto thinking about intellectual disability and being human, and more generally, as Wolff (2002: 123) suggests, Marx assumes 'that it is possible to be a universal human being in a particular sense, at least in post-capitalist society', so that when there are no longer economic divisions, 'we will be left with fellow-feeling for all human beings which transcends barriers of race, religion, nationality', and one might add gender, disability, sexuality and so on. This has not panned out, and we are not in a post-capitalist society. Yet we ought surely to address some of the issues that Marx proposed, and others continue to discuss, based on the fact that such oppression and dehumanisation is evident today. In this case, therefore, I will now look at Marx's theory of alienation and relate the different facets to everyday dehumanising and disabling experiences.

1 Alienation – from object of production

We lose sense of what it means to produce anything meaningful. For example, I used to work in a factory while I was studying. My relationship with what I was producing was meaningless. Coffee caps and toothpaste tube lids were made in the factory and then sent elsewhere. These objects were alien to me. Machines did the bulk of the work, yet as I stood on the factory line, unable to move due to the fact that if I did the boxes would overflow, I lost some of my humanness and behaved like a machine. This seems dated, yet as an intellectually disabled person unable to contribute to production at many levels, unable to move, figuratively and sometimes literally, there is a sense of distance from human worth and dignity that could be expressed through the term alienation.

2 Alienation – in the act of production

What we do belongs to someone else, usually our employer. It is not part of our being, so therefore we cannot necessarily feel good about it, as in the instance of producing food and goods for self-sufficiency. Or with a tweak, in more contemporary and personal terms, feeling good about delivering lectures and carrying out research (despite them belonging to the employer) are also part of academic identity, being human and production. But for many, there is no choice; for example, back to when I was working in a factory, I was forced to work, not *literally* but I was a lone mother with a disabled daughter, studying, with a need to put food on the table and keep a roof over our heads. My activity belonged elsewhere – to someone else. If an intellectually disabled person is unable to have this relationship to production (or requires advocacy) due to their impairments, again, a sense of human worth diminishes in this context.

3 Alienation – from species being (so what makes us human, rather than animal?)

We become estranged from our self, from our humanness. In a capitalist society we no longer feel at one with our own spirit. Our ideas, plans and hopes are no longer a part of our essence, our being. For sure, we are a long way into capitalism, but how we might understand this is to consider how public sector workers might feel in their work, as political systems change and develop within neoliberalism. For example, my father, a social worker and left-wing Labour Party member, in the 1960s, '70s and '80s saw his species being drained away. His humanness became more automated, his work more bureaucratic, so much so that he took early retirement on the grounds of mental ill health (and burnout). The point is that we might meet our physical needs, but what about our emotional needs? Our emotional needs ought to be met, regardless of our cognitive ability. Moreover, our emotional (and identity development) needs can be met by working in paid employment, as seen below in a personal example about my daughter and her employment.

4 Alienation – from each other, human to human

This is probably the most significant aspect of alienation when talking about intellectual disability and being human, largely because we are estranged from each other, not in a Hegelian sense, but as a result of modern capitalist society. We no longer interact with each other as one human to another, we lack care and concern for others in an interactive and relational way. We are care-less. Arguably, we could say we care, from a distance (so caring about rather than for), for example, when pledging money as a result of a mass telethon, but is this really caring, is it ethical caring and care-full and does it involve compassion? I suggest not. This caring from a distance could be described as alienating. The 'tragic' stories of disabled, poverty-stricken children and families are on the one hand brought to life on the television screen, and yet they are in many ways 'faceless' distant stories, used to provoke emotion. But only enough to produce a tear or two, and trigger financial gift-giving. Moments later, and after feeling guilt for living a 'tragedy-free' life is satiated, we forget, deny, and move on: equilibrium is restored. *This alienation in current capitalist society is the most sinister in our understanding of being human and intellectual disability.*

Despite alienation, there are caring and care-full spaces too, with some humanity, which one might consider. I wrote this on my Facebook page in June 2015:

> Good Stuff! As some are aware (daughter) works at a franchise in Debenhams. She works four hours a week (two hours two mornings). To (daughter) this is a fundamental part of being a human being, contributing to society and earning a wage (albeit it is 'spends' not food and life money!). The past two weeks have been very unsettling for her (and

several conversations with a regional manager for me). There has been a process of 'restructuring' across the country, and we all know this means for many, redundancies. She has had her third and final meeting today and although her days have changed she has kept her hours. The official letter she got two days ago said she and her colleagues were at risk of redundancy, so when I got home Wed night she was upset when I read her the letter. We are chuffed to bits she has kept her hours, and this also suggests (franchise) did right by her. It would have been very very easy to lose (daughter) given that she is not 'multi-skilled'. Also when they sent home the choice of hours and days she had there were only two slots of two hours. Our branch was the only one to do this, as usually people have a minimum of four hours (which [daughter] tried but it was hard for her to concentrate for so long). So clearly they were for her. BUT some colleagues have lost hours so could have picked those two hour slots to make up their hours. I don't know the ins and outs, but I am very proud of (daughter) for doing bril in the meetings (she even asked 'will I still get paid' and 'can I still take Friday off for the show in December!'). Go girl. I also am chuffed that (franchise) and her colleagues enabled this to happen at times of uncertainty.

For my purposes here with respect to Marx, and in the rest of this book, while all four aspects of Marx's theory of alienation have meaning in discussing intellectual disability, it is the latter two that resonate the most in moving away from the social model of disability and in grasping being human. Furthermore, how we comprehend this is in the context of care-less and care-full spaces, care ethics, capabilities and a politics of difference.[1] Therefore, I propose that capitalist society has had an alienating impact upon humanity, and, without a caring revolution and reform in political systems, we are all doomed and have lost all sense of humanness. I argue that this is the case, especially when considering some of the stories in the following chapters. I propose that by taking a care ethics position, as well as by exploring capabilities via Nussbaum, a platform where critical debate can take place is apparent. This is as a result of how I understand being human in relation to care, ethics, and relational circumstances. I am not simply mapping a social context, although that's important, largely because intellectually disabled people's impairments impact upon and are impacted by all spheres: the emotional, practical and socio-political. Also I assume that the social model has not gone far enough in eradicating oppressive and disabling barriers for intellectually disabled people. Moreover, I do not want to suppose that care ethics and rights positions are unable to communicate, despite clearly being at odds. I am, however, privileging care ethics, whilst making room for a positive critique of a rights/justice based discourse.

In a way, what I am attempting to do here is to understand being human and intellectual disability from a position that does not comfortably sit within a rights-based position, for example, within the context of intellectual disability and dependence: interdependence is the key. We are all interdependent. But crucially it is not sufficient just to say we are all interdependent as human beings, as it might relinquish socio-political or legal responsibility (Herring, 2013). It is clear from the narratives in this volume that intellectually disabled people are not always able to make choices, participate in social life, nurture relationships, contribute to learning in any traditional sense, and so on, and I would oppose those who suggest that all humans can position themselves within this particular narrative. Intellectually disabled people, and their close personal ties, have a particular position where, whilst gendered, classed and 'raced' discourses have a part to play, intellectual capacity further oppresses, discriminates, and penalises intellectually disabled people and their caring practices and relationships.

Without a care ethics model of disability that incorporates and critiques the three spheres of caring work – the *emotional*, where love and care are psycho-socially interrogated, the *practical*, where day-to-day care is carried out, and the *socio-political*, where social intolerance and aversion to difficult differences are played out – it will be difficult to find a way forward in understanding the lives of intellectually disabled people. Moreover, caring and being cared for might be considered as being outside of production in any meaningful way. If we consider this to be the case, humanity has lost all sense of humanness. If this is the case we all have to cooperate. In thinking about production and capitalism, Levitas (2001: 451) identifies a parallel between exclusionary and underclass debates including the 'unemployable'. These debates are important on two accounts when considering care and a care ethics model of disability. One, because family members who are unable to gain paid employment due to their additional caring commitments are positioned as less than human, and two, unemployment is dehumanising in current political and social conditions.

This inhumane and care-less position was increased by Gordon Brown's new deal in 2009 for 'making work pay', which targeted lone parents, the long-term unemployed and disabled people. Disability has been further targeted for spending cuts as the past coalition government's Spending Review announced:

> 12 per cent reduction in the Department for Education's non-schools budget (this covers all children's services funded by the Government) [and] 28 per cent decrease in local council allocations over the next four years (this includes funding for disabled children's services locally). Effectively this has meant less money for disabled children's services.
>
> (DfE, 2010)

Since the Conservative Party won the election in the UK in 2015, disabled people have been hit hard due to austerity measures that have seen the withdrawal of the Independent Living Fund and moves to axe the Disability Living Allowance (Utting, 2015). These changes impact in numerous ways, but the following seem pertinent here.

- Intellectually disabled adults are likely to be unemployed and are therefore marginalised or excluded from being full citizens based on their unemployed/poor status. This impacts all caring spheres and indeed is a care-less space within the socio-political sphere.
- Inclusion directives and policies, as well as privileging academic attainment, directly affect the education of intellectually disabled children, those caring with them and education professionals.

The impact of the Conservative government in 2015, austerity measures and a care-less way of positioning those 'in need' as those who are a danger to the social fabric of society is something that requires urgent appeal.

By taking a care ethics position, as well as exploring human capabilities and flourishing, I have found a platform where critical debate can take place, which is the result of understanding being human in relation to ethics, caring and justice. Furthermore, the broader psycho-social and socio-legal responses that feed into and out of the socio-political sphere need to be addressed via social relations in a caring and just manner, ethically. Notably, intellectually disabled people (and in particular contexts those who are in caring relations with them) are not always able to make choices, participate in social life, nurture relationships, contribute to learning in any traditional sense, or be economically independent: 'Caring easily disappears from the picture when the production of economic value becomes a national obsession' (Herring, 2013: 1). These contexts, along with the foundation of the three spheres of caring work and relations, are the starting point for a care ethics model of disability. Importantly, as Oliver (1990: 133) stated about disabled people a quarter of a century ago, 'the wind is indeed blowing; the direction that wind takes will depend upon more than just disabled people themselves'. It is time for all to address intellectual disability in a more caring, care-full and politically challenging way.

Grounding a care ethics model of disability: feminist ethics of care[2]

I turn my attention now to a feminist ethics of care in an attempt to position a care ethics model of disability, not least because, as Virginia Held suggests,

> Prospects of human progress and flourishing hinge fundamentally on the care that those needing it receive, and that the ethics of care stresses the moral force of the responsibility to respond to the needs of the dependent. Many persons will become ill and dependent for some periods of their later lives, including frail in old age, and some who are permanently disabled will need care the whole of their lives. *Moralities built on the image of the independent, autonomous, rational individual largely overlook the reality of human dependence and the morality for which it calls.*
>
> (Held, 2006: 10, emphasis added)

Indeed, there is a growing body of literature which marks out and endorses a feminist ethics of care, and critiques established ways of thinking about ethics, compassion, morality, citizenship, security, and care. It also provides alternatives in mapping these, as it operates at an epistemological and theoretical level, but also at the level of practical application (Sevenhuijsen, 2003). This is why it would seem appropriate for me to propose a care ethics model of disability. Certainly I could consider a socio-political model or a psycho-social model, aspects of which would be suitable in considering being human and intellectual disability, or I might explore a justice/rights version, which would largely be developed via a social model of disability. However, a care ethics model, like the social model, interrogates political and relational implications, yet specifically draws from caring and ethical relations. Moreover, unlike the social model (and areas of ethics of care), a care ethics model is not about the removal of social barriers *per se*, as this on its own is insufficient for intellectually disabled people. After all, severely intellectually disabled people will not be rid of everyday oppression, prejudice and danger if relationships (emotional, practical, and socio-political) are not reconceptualised beyond the social/ institutional level. The psycho-social and cultural aspects of human interaction too need to be remodelled and reconceptualised.

The care ethics model of disability is about trust and webs of relationships, and focuses on both the receiver and the giver of care (Tronto, 2011). It is not about individual rights and freedom, as this detracts from the politics of care and leads us to a paternalistic state of doing and being, where those who are considered more vulnerable, frail and dependent are placed in a powerless position. We ought not to forget that human flourishing is part of being human, and that this, one could argue, is individually driven. I, and other feminist ethics of care writers, would suggest that flourishing is always relational. Critically, intellectually disabled people are always interdependent, and many would not survive without a caring other(s). Removing social barriers without fully committing to a moral, political and ethical formulation of caring is not an option; care and caring can no longer be seen as a private matter. Robinson (2011a: 29) says many things about feminist care ethics, but notably interrogates human security. I, however, would like to focus on the idea that there is a commitment to moral issues, particularly in relation to real lived experiences, and a reconceptualisation of how we understand the public and private spheres. It is clear in the following chapters that real lived experiences, explored via narrative research and personal reflection, are central to grasping a care ethics understanding, but, for now, I will briefly map a feminist ethics of care.

Spanning over 30 years, feminist ethics of care literature can loosely be divided into two waves, with Carol Gilligan and Nel Noddings as central figures in the early 1980s, suggesting, crucially for my work, that 'an ethic of justice proceeds from the premise of equality – that everyone should be treated the same – an ethic of care rests on the premise of nonviolence' (Gilligan, 1993: 174) and that 'the loveliest of human functions, depends upon and interacts with dialogue and practice' (Noddings, 2003: 196).[3] Certainly, as we begin to understand the lives of intellectually disabled people and those who interact with them, we grasp that equality does not mean the same for everyone, but that non-violence is an expectation we can and should assume. It is also important that within the emotional, practical and socio-political spheres we anticipate a caring dialogue and practice.

Some of these earlier key thinkers in feminist ethics of care including Nel Noddings (2003), Sara Ruddick (1989) and Joan Tronto (1987, 1993a) composed accounts of the particular relationship between women and ethics of care. This often involved a consideration of the mother–child relationship as a specific and significant example of the intertwining of ethics and everyday life. Whilst the embodied aspects of motherhood are fully recognised, it is the gendering of the social roles of women, and indeed of morality, which are emphasised, producing accounts of moral reasoning which are grounded in, but not limited to, women's experiences of care. When thinking about the cases and narratives included in this book I have focused on aspects of everyday life that impact upon intellectually disabled people and those caring with and for them, whether that is in response to family caring, education, professionals' caring, or personal and intimate relations. From this perspective, and via these contexts, care is understood and presented as a practice and as a way of thinking. Yet, often within these areas of 'caring' I discover care-less spaces that damage, thwart, and contest caring work. Indeed, within these spaces human beings are in danger. The development of a feminist ethics of care has sought to define care in more grounded terms, but also, at a philosophical level, it has aimed to reposition and argue for the value of care as a basis for moral and political theory and also for social policy. Importantly too, in thinking beyond the persona and into the socio-political sphere, I have already identified care-less media representations that demonstrate the broader context of caring. Here, social justice and care ethics, mass systemic (and sometimes actual) violence are recognised.

Significantly, Noddings' (2003) work is important in the conceptualisation of care and caring as a starting point for an alternative moral theory, and offers a detailed definition of care as a central, crucial and *human* practice. She presents, as do others (for example Ruddick, 1989), care as a practice and therefore as learnt and, importantly, as improvable, but also argues that experiences of being cared for are definitively human, or 'universally accessible' (Noddings, 2003: 5). This point illustrates a significant theme in feminist ethics, which is to highlight the commonality of human vulnerability, not just at the beginning and end of life but as a constant and fundamental condition. Actually this point is vital to understanding intellectual disability, because we all need care at some point, and are all therefore interdependent. Yet this also must not be used as, or considered to be, a reason not to provoke more nuanced ways of caring with other humans, who are clearly less able. We cannot *simply* say we will all need care at some point in our lives (cradle to grave), as the shades of difference in this interpretation are significant. Essentially here,

Noddings presents a central relationship between the 'one-caring' and the 'cared-for', arguing that while a relationship involves both parties, more often than not, the one-caring is practically doing more work. It is neither symmetrical nor equal, yet those who are 'cared for' are always seen as contributing. The relationship between those caring and those cared for is seen as having important implications for developing a feminist moral theory which does not relegate or romanticise women's experiences of care, and which does not reduce caring to a selfless or self-sacrificial act. Yet when we read and research about what happens for families and intellectually disabled people, we might critique whether this is indeed happening. Related to this, Noddings distinguishes between 'natural caring', which she sees as spontaneous and most evident within the mother–child relationship, and caring as an 'ethical ideal', which refers to the process by which we struggle to reason, act and relate to others in an ethical way. Noddings also makes a distinction between 'caring for', which she sees as involving caring activities and responsibilities experienced directly, and 'caring about', which involves a more indirect concern and potential for caring activity with those at greater distance. That said, this conceptualisation of care ethics forms the basis for the recognition and valuing of caring work and caring relations, and provides an important platform for the notions of interdependence and a relational self (Robinson, 2011a; Sevenhuijsen, 1998; Tronto, 1993a).

Arguably, Tronto and Sevenhuijsen form the core of a second wave from the early 1990s onwards. This engagement with care ethics has continued to develop across a number of disciplines, including Sociology, Geography, Psychosocial Studies, Philosophy and Social Policy, and there has been particular interest from those studying family lives and relationships (Doucet, 2006; Duncan and Edwards, 1999; Ribbens McCarthy, Edwards and Gillies, 2003; Smart and Neale, 1999). Here a focus has been on revealing the moral and ethical aspects of family lives and extending the range of contexts in which caring relations and responsibilities are seen to exist and are struggled with. Tronto and Fisher (1990) offer a slightly different, broader definition of caring than that of Noddings:

> A species activity that includes everything that we do to maintain, continue and repair our 'world', so that we can live in it as well as possible. That world includes our bodies, ourselves, and our environment, all of which we seek to interweave in a complex, life-sustaining web.
>
> (Tronto and Fisher, 1990: 40)

They set out what they describe as four aspects of care: caring about, taking care of, care giving and care receiving. All four are important and relevant when disentangling education, mothering and intimacy. Alongside these are corresponding ethical values: attentiveness, responsibility, competence and responsiveness, each of which also act as evaluative criteria, producing both the possibility for considering good enough caring, and for defining moral or ethical failings, such as 'inattentiveness' or 'privileged irresponsibility'. Tronto and Fisher (1990) also define these ethical values from the premise of a connected, relational and socially situated self, and that of care as a practice with both cognitive and affective elements, rather than constructing or drawing on notions of abstract and formal moral principles. This concern with developing a moral theory grounded in context and practice, and emphasising the process of moral deliberation and decision making rather than a detached conformity to absolute moral rules, is, again, a central preoccupation of writers in this field. A number of recurring debates have emerged in the process of seeking to reposition and enrich understandings of care. Three of these – the value of care for moral and political theory, the relationship between care and gender, and that between justice and care – are directly relevant to some of the cases discussed in this book.

Importantly, Sevenhuijsen's (1998: 6) work shares with Tronto's (and that of others) an interest in 'a search for an appropriate vocabulary for making care into a political issue from a feminist perspective'. The focus of Sevenhuijsen's work, more specifically, has been to explore and argue for the value of care in relation to citizenship; again seeking to critique traditional models of both the citizen and the nature of citizenship. I would argue that this is a starting point, but that the idea of citizenship is also wrapped up in what it means to be human within any community. Sevenhuijsen also asserts that a feminist ethics of care can offer not only new ways of thinking about citizenship as an aspect of ethical life, but also about morality itself and the process of 'judging'. And again, this morality and judgement is significant in intellectual disability research as we begin to map how differently able others are placed along a spectrum of ability – where they can be judged and morally assessed.

Alongside the re-valuing of women's experiences of caring, there is also the aim of critiquing the gendered, unequal distribution of caring labour and seeking to establish care as a central social and political issue. In this way then, the literature on a feminist ethics of care provides another example of a much wider and longstanding feminist concern with pursuing equality *without equating this to sameness* (Sevenhuijsen, 2000: 28). Importantly for this book, concerns about the relationship between caring and justice in relation to intellectual disability are prioritised. Since Gilligan's initial proposal of an alternative ethic of care, two core ideas, of care and justice, have been contrasted:

> An ethic of justice focuses on questions of fairness, equality, individual rights, abstract principles, and the consistent application of them. An ethic of care focuses on attentiveness, trust, responsiveness to need, narrative nuance and cultivating caring relations.
>
> (Held, 2006: 3–4)

Much attention has been paid to questions about the nature and extent of differences between justice and care (see recent critiques, Robinson, 2011a,

2011b; Tronto, 2011) and the implications of such differences in terms of the epistemological, cultural and practical value of each. If justice and care are seen to be oppositional then the ethics of care must either be convincingly presented as a preferable or superior alternative, or risk being relegated to a secondary positioning.

For writers such as Tronto, this risk is associated particularly with what she sees as 'feminine' accounts of an ethics of care: 'As long as women's morality is viewed as different and more particular than mainstream moral thought, it inevitably will be treated as a secondary form of moral thinking' (Tronto, 1993b: 246). If an ethics of care is seen as a replacement for an ethics of justice, then this could be detrimental to the pursuit of equality; a conception and language of 'rights' has long been a resource for those challenging prejudice and discrimination. An alternative strategy is to see justice and care as, in some ways and to some extent, compatible or integrated, and that both may be necessary for a systematic theory of morality and ethics. A care ethics model of disability incorporates both caring and justice. However, there are a number of significant issues involved in attempting to reconcile or combine caring and justice, such as the conception and evaluation of needs. Part of exploring the extent to which care and justice perspectives may share common concerns or contain elements of one another has been to consider the kinds of moral questions they ask, or the moral problems they raise. One such question, as identified by Tronto (1993a), is how best to understand human 'needs' and how competing needs may be evaluated and met. I have already indicated that needs are a critical aspect to consider when thinking about caring and intellectual disability. Tronto offers a critical consideration of the conception of need, arguing that a care perspective may offer a more appropriate means of understanding, and judging, complex human needs. For example, she argues that a traditional model of justice concerning rights-bearing individuals tends to reduce or alienate those deemed 'needy', presenting a skewed and inaccurate picture of the characteristics of both the people themselves and their needs. Because the ethics of care foregrounds human vulnerability and the need for care, where care is seen as relating to material, emotional and psychological well-being, Tronto (1993a) argues that it not only incorporates justice questions, but is equally, if not better, placed to respond to them. This is certainly pertinent for intellectual disability research.

This concern with asserting the relevance of care to issues of justice and equality is one that has continued in feminist care ethics, political philosophy, law and sociology over the past two decades. It has been articulated in terms of 'affective inequality' (Lynch, Baker and Lyons, 2009), 'interdependency and caringscapes' (Bowlby et al., 2010), 'species membership' (Nussbaum, 2006), caring and the law (Herring 2013), and 'human security' (Robinson, 2011a). These works assert the general arguments that all human societies require the provision of love and care, that interdependency is the 'condition' of human beings, and that love and care cannot be understood without recognition of the 'gendered order of caring' (Lynch, Baker and Lyons, 2009: 219). So, in light of the reinvigoration of debates on care by the likes of Barnes (2006), Bowlby and her colleagues (2010), Lynch and her colleagues (2009), Robinson (2011a, 2011b) and Mahon and Robinson (2011), the relevance of care for political and policy responses to social and economic inequalities, and in particular intellectual disability, is apparent. This is further evidenced in Robinson's (2011a) work within political philosophy and international relations discussing human security. She argues that we are beings-in-relation and maps the importance of networks of relations along with challenging assumptions about dependency and vulnerability. These points are critical in understanding intellectual disability, especially for this book as we move through education, mothering and intimacy, all of which employ networks of relations. It is also critical to grasp the fact that not only do institutions and relationships work together – home, school, community, friends, hospital, family, government, carers, professionals, charities – but they all, in principle, feed into and out of each other, which is why a care ethics model of disability is useful. And that which was once private (care), for example, is now a public matter (Robinson, 2011a; Wright Mills, 1959).

This idea of care being public is not just about the public in the socio-political sphere (wider public and bureaucracy), although this is important and something I will discuss further, but about care, caring and relationality being the guiding principles of care ethics and morality. So being human is not simply about the autonomous individual, as Noddings describes: 'To be with another in time of trouble is better than to be permanently alone and trouble free [...] One loses both the "human" and the "being" when one is severed from all relation' (Noddings, 2003: 174). What is evident from available research is that intellectually disabled children and adults are often left alone, without caring relations, whether that is in a locked ward, in supported living, in 'care', in hospital, or even in school (see Rogers, in press). Many do not often experience caring relations and this works against human security. Robinson's (2011a) work positions human security within a feminist ethics frame and suggests that the key to this new understanding is that individual human rights, while relevant, are inadequate as a normative and analytic basis. Indeed, by 'foregrounding and prioritizing the consideration of politics of care, we can recover the potential of human security to focus attention on innovative strategies for addressing exclusion and oppression that are neither Western-centric nor imperialistic' (Robinson, 2011a: 14).

Significantly, Robinson looks at care, humanity and social justice in different global contexts and institutions, under the banner of human security. She draws on the fact that human security emerged as an idea in the early 1990s when historical, academic and policy developments came together in an unusual convergence. Moreover, it was thought that the human individual ought to be the chief recipient of the outcomes of 'security policy and security analysis' (Robinson, 2011a: 46). Broadly speaking, it is, as she refers to Newman, a '"freedom from want" and "freedom from fear"' (Robinson, 2011a: 47). But Robinson is dissatisfied with the way human security has been developed, as it is clear that everybody would want to feel secure but very few people understand what it actually means. I am unable to go into the detailed history of how Robinson maps human security but note that from this conceptual understanding considered within a feminist ethics of care, as I have noted, the self is relational, we are all interdependent, and care is *not* a private matter anymore. These things come together in developing a care ethics model of disability, via the three spheres of caring. Therefore, to feel secure, and indeed safe, in being human, we might understand this via institutions and relationships as Robinson suggests. In the following chapters, I engage with institutions and relationships via the family, carers, intimacy, friendships, school, home and community, for example. A feminist ethics of care is useful, but casting the net a little wider, I argue that a care ethics model of disability can be facilitated by exploring the work of Martha Nussbaum.

Capabilities and being human

There are some significant clashes between a feminist ethics of care and Nussbaum's (2000, 2004, 2006, 2011) work generally, not least because feminist ethics of care approaches are non-Kantian and non-rights based, in essence. However, as I interrogate being human and intellectual disability, I would like to focus on capabilities, as I consider this holds some significance in conceptualising the emotional, practical and socio-political caring spheres within a care ethics model of disability. Therefore I ought not to dismiss social justice and human rights discourse without significant discussion. As it is, John Vorhaus (2016: 38) recommends looking to human capabilities in his philosophical work on profound and multiple disability, yet argues that the 'concept of "capability" cannot be so elastic as to allow us to conclude that all human beings are similarly endowed with capabilities, irrespective of impairment, disability and other facts about us'; indeed, he goes on to say 'there is more to what is valuable about a person, including what they can offer other people, than is likely to be revealed in an audit of their capabilities and functionings' (Vorhaus, 2016: 38–39). That said, it is worth recognising Amartya Sen (2009) as hugely influential in understanding inequality and human development, but here I take a more in-depth look at Nussbaum and her work around capabilities.

Undeniably, Nussbaum (2011) suggests the 'capabilities approach' is a political, not moral, doctrine about basic entitlements. Moreover, it largely responds to and engages with social contract theory and Utilitarianism in offering something that can be presented as a type of human rights approach (Nussbaum, 2006). Inspired by Rousseau's 'profound contention that political equality must be sustained by an emotional development that understands humanity as a condition of shared incompleteness' (Nussbaum, 2004: 16), and drawing on S. J. Mill generally, Nussbaum understands that 'just institutions, if they are to be stable, require support from the psychology of citizens' and '[i]nstitutions must be sustained by the good will of citizens, but they also embody and teach norms of what a good and reasonable citizen is'

(Nussbaum, 2004: 16). She emphasises the need for decent living conditions and a creative space, which must include the potential for human beings to do what they want and be who they want to be (Nussbaum, 2011), as she asks '[w]hat real opportunities are available to them?' (Nussbaum, 2011: x). These points are the premise of Nussbaum's (2011) capabilities approach.

I cannot argue with this, in principle, but when we begin to mine intellectual disability research and experiences of caring the question arises, 'what real opportunities are available to each human?' Here I might distinguish between the carer (the one caring) and those cared for/with/about. This is deeply problematic. Yet, simply because I might have a problem in philosophically fusing care ethics and rights at a foundational level, do I dismiss Nussbaum's insightful work? It might be there is a way of thinking and understanding the social world in a more pluralistic way. For example, as Ken Plummer, in the context of sexualities, suggests

> The world in which we live is a 'pluralistic universe'. And human sexualities, like human life, are born of these pluralities. Even as we live under the dominance of singular coercive states trying to create singular hegemonic order, we still live plural lives in plural cultures with plural values, religions, politics, identities and affiliations, as well as plural genders and plural sexualities. By plural, I highlight multiplicities, difference and variety. *Human beings cannot help this plurality: it is surely one of the things that makes us human.*
>
> (Plummer, 2015: 13; emphasis added)

In being human, and in understanding caring, it seems critical to understand caring relations and practices as pluralistic. As it is, in his previous work over a decade ago, Plummer asked the questions: 'how can we find some sense of the universal, however limited among all the pluralisation, polyvocality, and difference?' and 'how will we live with a postmodern ethics that recognizes the importance of "freedom, justice, equality, care, recognition, minimal harm"?' (Plummer, 2003). Clearly his work has moved on, but in essence the thread of interrogating social phenomena in a diverse and varied manner is still evident. With respect to, in his case sexualities and in my case intellectual disability, the idea that we can simply sit with one viewpoint and understand complex human interaction and relations is narrow-minded and ultimately restrictive in progressing knowledge and practice.

Therefore, I propose that Nussbaum, in her recent volumes, has much to add to a critical understanding of intellectual disability and humanity, and consider this work within my proposed care ethics model of disability, particularly within the socio-political sphere. As the capabilities approach is about basic entitlements, and sets up ways of thinking about, and then potentially making a difference within, political, social and economic contexts, it seems sensible at least to address this position as social intolerance and aversion to difficult differences are played out. For Nussbaum (2006) if we do not follow the capabilities approach we are in danger of promoting a life without dignity (or worth), and indeed dignity is essential for human flourishing and development (see also Stienstra and Ashcroft, 2010). Importantly for intellectually disabled people, any 'decent society must address their needs for care, education, self-respect, activity, and friendship' (Nussbaum, 2006: 98). Therefore I suggest we ought to enter into this debate in order to enable interdependence, gain social justice and make people listen – within a relational and care ethics context. In truth, a just, care-full and ethical society would not hinder the development of, access to, and engagement with education, social support, work, relationships and unprejudiced representation for intellectually disabled people, their families and those caring. A just, care-full and ethical society would not exclude, marginalise or oppress anyone (Hartley, 2009; Hull, 2009a, 2009b; Wolff and De-Shalit, 2007). It would support a participatory and meaningful existence in all areas of life, including education, relationships and political life (whatever guise that might take). The caring involved needs to be non-exploitative and it is here that a care ethics model would exist via the emotional, practical and socio-political spheres, in a relational, care-full and ethical way, rather than simply with respect to rights otherwise there will always be losers, whether that is the one caring or those cared for/with/about.

Importantly, Nussbaum (2006), in her thesis on justice, draws on classical theory much of the time, and says that those being 'spoken to' via the social contract, for example, were men. Others, namely women, children and the elderly, were not seen as economically productive and were therefore excluded from this discourse and from full participation in civil society. A great deal of this exclusion in recent history has been resolved *to an extent*, but no 'social contract doctrine, however includes people with severe and atypical physical and mental impairments in the group of those by whom basic political principles are chosen' (Nussbaum, 2006: 15). To this end, institutions, especially educational establishments, 'must be sustained by the good will of citizens, but they also embody and teach norms of what a good and reasonable citizen is' (Nussbaum, 2004: 16). I understand that Nussbaum emphasises the need for decent living conditions and a creative space and this must include that human beings are able to do and be who they want to be (Nussbaum, 2011), as she asks what 'real opportunities are available to them?' (Nussbaum, 2011: x). This is a crucial question to thinking about a meaningful life for all, not just intellectually disabled people, especially as human rights *per se* can be problematic and work against social conscience. Human rights for all means someone will suffer – the one caring, the cared for/about/with. I am attempting to make sense of this here.

In considering Nussbaum's position, it is worth identifying her ten central capabilities (Nussbaum, 2011: 33–34) which must be enabled to ensure a dignified and minimally flourishing life, as human flourishing is essential in being human.

1 *Life*: not dying prematurely, or living a life not worth living.
2 *Bodily health*: having good health (including reproductive health), shelter and food.

3   *Bodily integrity:* freedom to move around, to be secure from any violence or abuse, and to have the opportunity to gain sexual pleasure and have reproductive choices.

4   *Senses, imagination, and thought*: being able to use the senses, think and reason.

5   *Emotions:* to be able to love, care, grieve, and show gratitude and justified anger. Not to have these thwarted for fear of anxiety.

6   *Practical reason:* being able to think about the good and reflect about one's life.

7   *Affiliation:*
    a   Live with and towards others and engage in social interaction.
    b   Have the social bases for self-respect and make provisions for non-discrimination.

8   *Other species:* concern for other non-human animals, nature and environment.

9   *Play:* being able to laugh, play and enjoy leisure.

10   *Control over one's environment:*
    a   Political: have the right to participate in political life.
    b   Material: have rights, seek work, hold property on an equal basis to others.

Nussbaum states, for example, that these central capabilities do not presume to solve all economically driven distribution problems, but at least propose a significant social minimum for a quality of life, and all ten are an essential condition of social justice (see Held, 1995 and Shakespeare, 2006, for other social justice discourses).[4]

I do not, however, think that there ought to be a social minimum, as this implies that we can put up with lack and care-less spaces. It also sets up a hierarchy of impairment, experience and control over one's environment which might work against interdependence in the grander scheme of things. Intellectually disabled people, and those caring, already have actual everyday restrictions to do with impairments, as well as disabling conditions. Notably, human rights approaches are closely aligned to the capabilities approach, and those focused upon core entitlements; so, for example, with a human rights position, the first generation of rights-based discourse was positioned within political and civil rights and the second generation towards economic and social rights (Nussbaum, 2011: 63). Just as legal discourse can be problematic in setting up binary positions (see Herring, 2013), so too can rights discourse. Being human within an intellectual disability context is far more complicated. The capabilities approach 'makes evident the complex forms of inter-dependence between human beings and their material, social and political environments' (Nussbaum, 2004: 345), and this way of thinking about and doing justice is 'well suited to provide the core for society that seeks to acknowledge humanness (including animality, mortality, and finitude) rather than to hide from it, calling shame and disgust to its aid' (Nussbaum, 2004: 345). One might therefore call for interdependence within a socially just society that is care-full – in other words, a care ethics model of disability. Or one might call for

> a society that acknowledges its own humanity, and neither hides us from it nor it from us; a society of citizens who admit that they are needy and vulnerable, and who discard the grandiose demands for omnipotence and completeness that have been at the heart of so much human misery, both public and private.
>
> (Nussbaum, 2004: 17)

Surely my proposal ought to include this acknowledgement? Nussbaum's (2011) *Creating Capabilities* is an overarching window into previous work focused on the capabilities approach, but it is not the only work that is relevant here in discussing ethics, caring and intellectual disability, as stated above. Indeed, it is simply a summary of the capabilities approach; yet this work is critical in thinking about what Nussbaum has said regarding disgust and shame. Moreover, the idea of dignity is a universal position that speaks to all nations and all humans. Nussbaum (2011) tends to use the capabilities approach generally in her work, but it is also known as the Human Development Approach.[5] This approach is suggested as a new paradigm[6] that is often associated with 'poorer', 'developing' countries such as India, based on the crude, it seems, measures of Gross Domestic Product (GDP) per capita, and quality of life. High GDP does not necessarily match with a quality of life for all; as we know, there are huge inequalities and injustices that cannot be measured sufficiently by simply looking at GDP. Therefore, making assumptions about human development, well-being and freedom based upon this measure is deeply problematic. It is also clear that problems relating to human development are not simply an issue for the global South, but that the global North too has inequities that are not insignificant when it comes to human development. So, from Nussbaum's position, she sees all countries as 'developing' in one way or another. The premise of capabilities, as I have implied already, is based on this question: 'What are people actually able to do and be? What real opportunities are available to them?' (Nussbaum, 2011: x). It might seem obvious that this simple premise is important in discussing being human and intellectual disability, based on the fact that so many intellectually disabled people are unable to do what they want and be who they want to be. Moreover, based on an intellectually disabled person's varying impairments, we might also consider those caring are also unable to do and be who they want to be. This is crucial in understanding a care ethics model of disability, as it is not a binary position. Doing and being who we want to be is always relational and interdependent, not with the State, but in relation to one another. This is why proposing a care ethics model of disability is critical, as the socio-political has a socially just and ethical job to do on a grander scale, yet it is still interdependent and relational with respect to the emotional and practical spheres.

As it is, much of Nussbaum's work has been based around theorising human development via the capabilities approach, drawing on and critically engaging with an array of economic and political philosophy from over the decades, as well as some sociological and psychological theory. She suggests, and I would agree, that theories are a 'large part of our world, framing the way issues are seen, shaping perceptions of salience, and thus slanting debate toward certain policies rather than others' (Nussbaum, 2011: xi). In a similar way to me, in understanding theory and philosophical positions, Nussbaum (2011) theorises stories throughout her work. For example, in *Creating Capabilities* she explains the capabilities approach largely through consideration of the experiences of Vasanti, a woman from north-western India. In a nutshell, Vasanti had an alcoholic husband who spent all the family money and had a vasectomy for a cash incentive, leaving her in poverty and childless. Her husband became more abusive and she left him. What Nussbaum is doing here is including the narratives as a way into the sometimes difficult and complex philosophical and social positions, so as to display and story human lives and social injustice, which then shows how public policy can make a difference.[7] She suggests that we look at life stories so that we can find the meaning in policy changes for real people (Nussbaum, 2011: 14), but recognises that story telling is 'never neutral' as the 'narrator always directs attention to some features of the world rather than to others' (Nussbaum, 2011: 15).

As such, regarding the capabilities approach, we are required to make clever policy choices and commit to action that enables people to be the best that they can be. Contractarianism and Utilitarianism, for example, are deep-rooted, yet Nussbaum has proposed a development theory that takes issue with the unjustifiable global problems for human beings, and demands that people deserve their dignity. As I have said, initially this approach was associated with the poorer nations and often discussed in relation to inter-inequity, or disparity between nations. However, it is increasingly recognising the intra-inequity in countries with high GDP and that people in the global North, in sometimes different ways, are living without dignity and are struggling to have quality of life. The capabilities approach (or Human Development Approach) is the key political/economic program that Sen (1992, 1999, 2009) has proposed in response to unsatisfactory evaluations in understanding and plotting quality of life for human subjects.

I have listed the capabilities above, but I want to identify further that Nussbaum argues capability is a 'kind of freedom' (2011: 20), and there are 'substantial freedoms' that she calls *combined capabilities*, which are the totality of opportunities for choice and action in one's specific political, social and economic circumstances (Nussbaum, 2011: 21). Then there are *internal capabilities* which are, for example, intellectual and emotional capacities, physical health and movement, skills of perception and more. She says that these are not necessarily fixed, but fluid and dynamic, and therefore not innate but often developed *or not.* Why is it necessary then to distinguish between the two? Importantly, on one hand, a 'society might do quite well at producing internal capabilities but might cut off avenues through which people actually have the opportunity to function in accordance with those capabilities' (Nussbaum, 2011: 21). So they may well gain an education and be able to express themselves politically but then be denied freedom of expression. Alternatively, which could be pertinent for intellectually disabled people, it might be 'possible for a person to live in a political and social environment in which she could realize an internal capability [...] but lack the developed ability to think critically or speak publically' (Nussbaum, 2011: 22).

There are *basic capabilities* too, but these need to be addressed with some caution. Even though many aspects of being human are indeed socially and culturally defined, from very early on in childhood, intellectual impairments can queer this somewhat. Parallels can be drawn to the fact that the social model of disability does not always feel adequate when making sense of intellectually disabled people's lives because the removal of barriers to inclusion, for example, does not take away day-to-day challenges that exist. What Nussbaum says about intellectually disabled people is that the goal ought to be 'for them to have the same capabilities as "normal" people' (Nussbaum, 2011: 24), even though it is likely that for some these will be expressed with or through an advocate. All of this sounds suspiciously similar to the social model, which as we know has become less and less relevant within areas of intellectual disability research and less and less relevant for the actual lives of those who are caring and are cared for/about/with. A feminist ethics position combined with a care ethics model is more convincing. Nonetheless there is human freedom in the capabilities approach, so not dictating that people must live healthy lives, pursue a particular religion and carry out certain activities. As Nussbaum has said, 'there is a huge moral difference between a policy that promotes health and one that promotes health capabilities' (Nussbaum, 2011: 26); capabilities are about respect for cultural, religious and lifestyle differences. There is a caveat here with children, as compulsory education is seen as a crucial introduction to adult capabilities. For example, for intellectually disabled people, I could suggest that inclusive education policies satisfy the need to educate everyone. (But this seems not be the case, as identified in the following chapter.) Yet in the main, as Nussbaum (2011: 30) suggests, 'we do not treat a child with Down Syndrome in a manner commensurate with that child's dignity if we fail to develop the child's powers of mind through suitable education'. In fact, for intellectually disabled people I might need to consider policies that support and care ethically and with interdependence rather than infantilise and 'treat them as passive recipients of benefit' (Nussbaum, 2011: 30).

Consequently, in the area of justice for intellectually disabled people, the Kantian elements of the social contract are problematic. This is because Kant 'grounds his respect on a high degree of moral rationality and thus is unable to accord fully equal respect to people with severe cognitive disabilities'

(Nussbaum, 2011: 85–86). Critically, Rawls' Kantian position is difficult to swallow as 'human beings who can't enter into agreements or contracts are not owed political justice' (Nussbaum, 2011: 87). This is largely down to rough equality and mutual advantage. So if humans are crudely equal and have a shared benefit, then all will be tolerable. This is not acceptable. The capabilities approach is therefore a form of political liberalism rather than a doctrine. Furthermore, education is seen as pivotal to the development and exercise of many other human capabilities (2011: 152), especially as illiteracy anywhere is *perceived* to be an enduring disability. Hence, for example, Sen says that famine is not just about a shortage of food (Nussbaum, 2011) just as Slee (2011) says that deaf education is not just about volume. I suggest intellectual disability is not *just* about inclusion and rights. I propose a scheme of social cooperation (Nussbaum, 2011: 150) that involves caring and care-full-ness: a care ethics model of disability.

In taking the capabilities approach and moving it forward through her work on 'disability, nationality and species membership' Nussbaum (2006) calls for an attempt to address three unsolved problems of social justice. These problems are: doing justice (for physically and intellectually disabled people); extending justice to all world citizens (the world as a whole); and dealing with the treatment of non-human animals (animals can suffer). The first two here are clearly relevant to the work of this book as justice for intellectually disabled people needs to be addressed globally, particularly in the areas of health, education, care and pleasure. The third 'problem' is less clear, due to the fact that making a distinction between a reasoning human being as a full 'normal' citizen and a human being who has the reasoning qualities of a non-human animal is deeply problematic legally, ethically and philosophically, but then animal rights activists have taken up this gauntlet as part of that challenge (Kittay and Carlson, 2010). Of course, all three are very important for this summary of work, but I am particularly interested in the first, as Nussbaum says disabled people

> are people, but they have not as yet been included, in existing societies as citizens on a basis of equality with other citizens. The problem of extending education, health care, political rights and liberties, and equal citizenship more generally to such people seems to be a problem of justice, and an urgent one.
>
> (Nussbaum 2006: 2)

For Nussbaum, this is a difficult one due to the fact that politically it requires new ways of thinking about social cooperation (rather than mutual advantage).[8] This requires a reshaping of theoretical structures rather than simply building on the old ones (Nussbaum, 2006: 2). These ideas around social justice can then be positioned within the capabilities approach, but, as I have argued, this ought to be from a care ethics model of disability, incorporating the three spheres of caring work.

Thinking then about social justice alone is problematic. Intellectually disabled people are not considered full citizens and they certainly struggle to get their voices heard, and at worst are dehumanised. The problem is when those in power make decisions based on attributes such as rationality, language, and roughly equal physical and mental capacity (Nussbaum, 2006: 16) as rudiments for participating in citizenship. This clearly excludes many intellectually disabled people from contributing to and participating in civil society. Basically, drawing on Hume,[9] to identify the extreme prejudice in classic theory 'the much weaker, whether in body or mind, are simply not part of political society, not subjects of justice' (Nussbaum, 2006: 49), and are therefore unable to fully participate in society for all intents and purposes as meaningful citizens. Nussbaum suggests therefore a basis of human capabilities as a source of political principles. These are the principles that underpin a liberal pluralistic society. Furthermore, human dignity and worth, discussed by Nussbaum, also aligns with Marx's body of work, as set out above.

Thinking further about the capabilities, every one of them means that life without them is a life without human dignity. The capabilities approach starts with the Aristotelian and Marxian perspectives on the human being as a social and political person in relation with others (Nussbaum, 2006: 85). This indeed resonates with my proposed care ethics model of disability, and a feminist ethics position as relational. As Aristotle said, 'it would be odd to imagine human beings flourishing outside of such relations' (cited in Nussbaum, 2006: 86). More importantly here, 'children and adults with mental impairments are citizens. Any decent society must address their needs for care, education, self-respect, activity, and friendship' (Nussbaum, 2006: 98). A just and ethical society would not hinder the development of disabled people; it would support caring inclusion in all areas of life, including political life. Meaningful caring for all, whether children, the elderly, or those who are ill or impaired, and a focus on support for the capabilities of life, health, and bodily integrity are the way forward (Nussbaum, 2006: 168). As it is, those caring (often mothers) lose out (Nussbaum, 2006: 170). Crucially a 'decent society will organise public space, public education, and other relevant areas of public policy to support such lives and fully include them, giving the caregivers all the capabilities on our list, and the disabled as many of them, and as fully, as is possible' (Nussbaum, 2006: 222).

There are important critiques of Nussbaum's work and the capabilities approach in relation to intellectual disability (Berube, 2010; Carlson and Kittay, 2010; Hartley, 2009; Stark, 2010; Terzi, 2007, 2009; Wolff, 2009), because Nussbaum draws from the social contract tradition. This is challenging because it cannot accommodate intellectual disability, due to the fact that agents are said to be independent, free and equal and are assumed to enter this 'contract' for mutual advantage. For intellectually disabled people and those caring for them 'this isn't a bug in the social-contract software – it's a feature of the program' (Berube, 2010: 99). Why then would anyone 'agree to create forms of social organization that will support and nourish some people who will never be capable of repaying the favor' (Berube, 2010: 99)? Nussbaum does address this in a few ways. She gets us to think about the life course and dependency (or interdependency, I would argue) from the cradle to the grave, although, as I have said, this is nuanced and complicated. Any theory of justice would need to take this on board and Nussbaum argues that as 'the life span increases, the relative independence that many people sometimes enjoy looks more and more like a temporary condition, a phase of life that we move into gradually and all too quickly begin to leave' (2006: 101). She goes on to say that anyone who imagines their life as complete and never in need of care is living in a fictional world when it comes to the characteristics of human life. Thus,

> care for children, elderly people, and people with mental and physical disabilities is a major part of the work that needs to be done in any society, and in most societies it is a source of great injustice. Any theory of justice needs to think about the problem from the beginning, in the design of basic institutional structure, and particularly in its theory of the primary good.
>
> (Nussbaum, 2006: 127)

This argument is not dissimilar to that of disability studies academics and disability activists, who argue that it is likely we will all be disabled at some point in life (see Davis, 2006; Swain et al., 2004; Thomas, 2007). 'Any theory of justice needs to think about the problem from the beginning, in the design of basic institutional structure, and particularly in its theory of the primary good' (Nussbaum 2006: 127). Therefore, if we have a theory of caring ethics and social justice from this perspective we need to understand what intellectual disability looks like when we consider differences and caring relations.

Caring and a care ethics model of disability

Caring has different meanings depending on context, and ultimately is all-encompassing. Furthermore, there is and ought to be an alternative to Kantian rights-based ethics. Within a care ethics model, via all three proposed caring spheres, human safety, relationships and caring are key. I have already identified that Robinson (2011a) interrogates human security by using a feminist approach to an ethics of care, and it is here I begin to see how the emotional, practical and socio-political spheres leak into and out of the private and public lives of humans (more often than not women) in complex ways. Moreover, all humans are in danger of violence and abuse, systemic or otherwise; indeed, as I have stated, care is no longer a private issue. The public domain, or the socio-political sphere, has to take into account all human beings. Besides, it is evident that philosophically, moral reasoning based on justice which 'asserts that morality is about the objective application of universalizable principles among mutually disinterested, disembodied individuals' (Robinson, 2011a: 5) is wholly unacceptable. We do not live in a world of abstraction; we live in a world of relationships, *in the real world*. The 'successful outing with the autistic child, or the happy haircut of the demented women' (Herring, 2013: 1) are not of interest to the rolling reporting of global economics, yet this is misguided. People are dependent on other people, always, and economics are reliant on caring practices.

Trying to understand social justice, ethics and morality from an 'objective' or homogenous standpoint is simply not helpful when plotting a care ethics model of disability. I agree with Robinson in her approach to an ethics of care, as she makes an ontological shift, 'one that allows us to see moral subjects as relational and to recognize ethics as fulfilling responsibilities through practices of care' (2011a: 28). In this way I can identify that we safeguard against pain, distress, suffering and exclusion, yet clearly it is insufficient simply to understand care work *per se*. Not only can policy implement critical changes for local and global care practices, but also how the law and legal systems respond. It is therefore also important to rethink the underlying values of the law, as for too long it has been 'arranged around the vision of an able, autonomous and unattached adult' (Herring, 2013: 2). Thus, when I think of how the *socio-political sphere* might map onto a care ethics model of disability I consider institutions and relationships as working together, just like human relations, and, broadly speaking, within policy and legal contexts. So 'institutions' such as families, schools, communities and hospitals are full of cultural and social norms, but they are not, in and of themselves, anything without the human being. We are friends, mothers, fathers, sons, daughters, carers, professionals, siblings and so on. Actually, politically, a feminist ethics of care 'seeks solutions to the problems of the giving and receiving of care that are nonexploitative, equitable, and adequate to ensure the flourishing of all persons' (Robinson, 2011a: 33).

Despite Robinson (2011a) setting her work within a human security frame, her intention is not to securitise care. However, she suggests that without webs of care and responsibility, in addition to a sense of security, caring will be impossible. It is through webs of relationships that a focus on freedom from fear and positive relational action, rather than human rights or absolute social justice-based tactics, will prove hopeful and beneficial within a care ethics model of disability. After all, 'rights alone may not be able to do the "moral work" that it needs to in order to provide a complete ethics' (Robinson, 2011a: 49). Life is messy, exhausting, and at times can be unbearable and cause human suffering, regardless of intellectual capacity and mental health (Craib, 1994; Nussbaum, 2004, 2006; Wilkinson, 2005). In addition, autonomous human beings are only autonomous *if* they are in safe and beneficial relations of care. Simply turning to the likes of Nussbaum (2004, 2011) and social justice-based arguments, or other rights-framed positions, rather than focusing on a care ethics and caring practices leave us in danger of paternalisation, where so-called autonomous and powerful others 'care' for those who are inferior. This is risky within care discourses generally, not least because care can rapidly become, as mentioned, benevolent paternalism (Robinson, 2011a). Therefore, the care ethics model of disability ought to take into consideration the caring spheres, the emotional, practical and socio-political, and be introduced in a way that is framed within a care ethics discourse, as it is based on webs or practices of care and is relational. All this considered, I then need to formulate routes to social justice that map onto intellectual disability via the spheres proposed. This means that social policy and the law can respond to dilemmas where everyone will be included, and, unlike rights-based positions, it is about all people being included within the spheres of caring, care-fully.

Indeed, as I have argued, there has been a move towards *and* beyond the social model of disability which has had a huge impact upon disabled people's lives. It seems that globally the medical model is often sanctioned as a popular way of thinking about disability (Allan, 2010b; Haller, Ralph and Zaks, 2010; Singal, 2010), especially with regards to education and the family. This is certainly a barrier to inclusion as it fails to see, for example, education (policy and practice) as in need of reform, therefore leaving the intellectually disabled child to be rendered problematic, and often excluded, within care-less spaces. This continued focus on the child (with apparent deficit) feeds a culture of blame, which can be further identified through neuroscience debates, even though families have additional and important knowledge about their child that can be tapped if a more community- (and communication-) based approach is sought (Hornby, 2010; McLaughlin et al., 2008; Rogers, 2007a, 2007b, 2011). Currently, policy discourses explicitly imply that parents are partners in the education process and yet this is not experienced by parents as such (Hodge and Runswick-Cole, 2008; Rogers 2011), and these discussions around parents and policy are not just a UK, or global North, issue but a problem to be dealt with globally, both practically and theoretically (Allan, 2010a; Alur, 2010; Nussbaum, 2006).

There is of course tension, largely based on the fact that not all humans start on an equal footing and, therefore, universal human rights as a catch-all are impossible to follow anyhow. Ultimately, I am a feminist positioning myself within a care ethics frame, but how that journey transforms and progresses is not straightforward in relation to discussing being human and intellectual disability. This is because I fundamentally believe we are relational as human beings. We want to be with people (Arendt, 1998; Noddings 2003), we interact, in whatever capacity, regardless of whether we have the intellectual/cognitive capacity to do so (Kittay, 2005, 2010). Experiencing carelessness, living in care-less spaces is emotionally, practically and politically 'a serious human deprivation for most people' (Lynch, Baker and Lyons, 2009: 1). Indeed, Robinson (2011a: 14) goes so far as to say that we need to foreground and prioritise a politics of care ethics so as to 'recover human security' because without care, human security suffers greatly. Whilst I agree with the positions about care, and the relational and ethics when discussing intellectual disability and being human, I also propose that we do not omit discussions about capabilities. Not because I follow the line that a rights-based approach is the way forward; I do not. This rights-based approach leaves us in a stagnating place, as we grapple with whose rights are more important, for example, in the case of the one caring and the one cared for. This position is piecemeal, where we consider the medical and social model of disability. Neither of these models wholly work for intellectually disabled people with respect to their contribution to, and participation in, the socio-political sphere, or indeed in their day-to-day social lives. I therefore need to deliberate how we go about changing and reworking caring in order to make meaning for intellectually disabled people.

Law, policy and the socio-political sphere: no place for emotions

Within a feminist ethics of care, humans are in relationships. In addition to this, all humans are vulnerable and therefore all can be both care givers and receivers. However, for Tronto (and others such as Herring, 2013: 57) *trust* is key, and given that care is often both 'physical and psychic intimacy, good care grows out of trust that develops among those giving and receiving care' (Tronto, 2011: 162–163). Tronto goes on to say that care 'creates a *relationship* among the parties caring and being cared for' and critically this 'relationship is not a "thing"' (Tronto, 2011: 163, emphasis in original). All human beings, via a care ethics model of disability, ought to commit to hearing what the seemingly less powerful have to say. Yet it is apparent that people do not listen, or hear, as demonstrated in the following chapters. As it is, many people deny any wrongdoing, lack a sense of responsibility (Cohen, 2001; Lefkowitz, 1998; Tronto, 2011), flee from obligation (Korsgaard, 1996, 2009), run from disappointment (Craib, 1994), and are care-less, so much so that it is understood those who are 'marked' or stigmatised are not equal, and are therefore in danger (see Goffman 1990). At the very least those identified as 'marked' are seen to exist at the bottom of the human hierarchy and only worthy of low-paid or un-paid work, for example. Tronto (2011) in her work is talking about women of colour in the USA, but with respect to intellectually disabled people and their caring relations, they too are marked. It is because intellectually disabled people are marked that a care ethics model is essential and a reorganisation and reframing of caring work proposed.

A care ethics model of disability must therefore be grounded within the emotional, practical and socio-political spheres of caring work and founded upon caring relations. These spheres cannot be separated out and completely understood individually (see Mahon and Robinson, 2011: 178). This is because, for example, how we understand and experience difficult differences is considered to be an emotional and personal response. If, for example, someone sees an obviously disabled couple getting intimate in public there may well be an internal conversation such as 'they ought not to do that in public', or 'eugh, what are they doing in a relationship' or 'aw, how sweet'. None of these responses are simply owned by the person; they are part of a much deeper psycho-social aversion to these difficult differences. That is not to say these responses are excusable, but they are bound up with, and part of, the socio-political, where cultural meanings about social norms are reproduced. That is, where social intolerance and aversion to difficult differences are played out.

To turn to an empirical example, I can demonstrate this in the education sector. A mother experiences exclusion in the playground because her son, who has attention deficit hyperactivity disorder (ADHD), is disruptive to his school peers and their education. Other mothers do not like the disruptive or difficult child, or indeed his mother. They both pose a danger; a danger to their 'regular', 'normal', unmarked children, to the equilibrium of the school and classes, to the teacher and other education professionals, to the delivery of the curriculum, to the playground antics, to maternal communication and so on (Rogers, 2007a, 2013c). All of these aspects of school life are part of the emotional, practical and socio-political. They feed into and out of each other, and intellectual disability, or social and behavioural difference, fractures and disturbs (Gillies, forthcoming). Socio-political narratives via policy directives, for example, that privilege academic excellence and promote an examination culture work against caring practices, where those who are not traditionally academically able are located. This in turn impacts upon how practically and emotionally we all engage with such everyday occurrences. Therefore, instead of focusing on such 'dangerous' people, who underline human vulnerability, lack of reason, and dependency, we all need to establish caring practices within a care ethics model of disability, where interdependence is privileged and 'care workers' are valued indiscriminately (Mahon and Robinson, 2011). This could be tricky considering that the legal system tends to have such power. It is in this context I would like to consider what Herring (2013) has to say about care ethics, as the socio-political sphere within the care ethics model of disability needs to work alongside the law.

As it is, the legal system struggles with anything that is not about autonomous individuals, and Herring (2013) suggests that we need to re-evaluate how those values underpinning the law are conceptualised. Rather than simply focusing on the individual and rights-based models, where often one person or organisation is pitched against another, we ought to recognise the significance of relational values. Herring explicitly draws upon care ethics in examining the law, and it is in this marriage between care ethics and law that I find the care ethics model of disability fits. But how does this work? After all, caring is a relational practice between two or more people. The law is best placed to deal with arguments and disputes, or, as Herring states, 'who did what to whom and when?' (2013: 2). Even if we do have disputes, social injustices and violence, such as in the cases we see in the following chapters, with the young intellectually disabled man who died in the bath, in care, the young intellectually disabled woman who was sexually assaulted by a gang, the mother who committed filicide, the young people left alone without friends, and exclusions from school – what do we do then? What do we do with the emotions? What do we do with these humans and care-less spaces?

As with other scholars engaging with care ethics, Herring (2013) argues that the premise the law focuses on is that of interdependent relationships rather than isolated individuals. As we understand, from the point of view of care ethics and intellectual disability research, caring is a basic human need and we cannot live without it if we wish to flourish as human beings. Herring (2013: 14), in his mapping of caring and the law, proposes four markers of care which are useful in understanding a care ethics model of disability within the emotional, practical and socio-political spheres. These markers are:

1   Meeting needs;
2   Respect;
3   Responsibility; and
4   Relationality.

According to Herring (2013) *meeting needs* is activity-based and he rejects that care is about a feeling, reminding us of Tronto's distinction between caring 'for' and caring 'about'. This caring 'about' as a feeling is certainly evident in relation to stories in the media and television representations, where I highlighted in the previous chapter regarding the human response to 'tragic' stories. Caring about someone by donating a sum of money, for example, is not the same as caring work within the practical sphere where day-to-day care work is carried out. The second marker of care is *respect*. Basically this is understood to be recognising the humanity in one another, listening to each other, carrying out work in a dignified manner, and being aware of the experience of care for another (Herring, 2013: 18–19). These are particularly relevant to a care ethics model of disability, and certainly within the emotional sphere. Respect is missing in so many of the narratives within this book from interpersonal lack to policy lack, and this is ultimately care-less.

Responsibility is the third marker of care for Herring (2013), and it is the acceptance of being responsible that is critical. Responsibility cuts across all spheres. Herring (2013: 20) is mindful to highlight, however, that just because we might identify two people as being in a responsible and caring relationship, this does not discount the obligation for others to intervene if a particular issue is noticed. The fourth marker of care is *relationality*. Herring (2013) is not saying care is relational and therefore all relationships are good, of course there are bad and abusive relationships, but that is not to say elements of the relationship lack care. This is why *respect* is central within his markers of care. Herring (2013: 24) does acknowledge that some critics might think his relationality marker overemphasises the 'rational and physical' parts of a relationship. For me, here, in understanding intellectual disability, he provides a good example of how this might not be the case, as someone who is profoundly intellectually impaired might be unable to reciprocate care in any traditional way, as a service. 'But relationships are made up of more than the doing of deeds and the saying of words. A touch, an expression, the slightest smile, can convey great warmth' (Herring, 2013: 24–25), and they are often fluctuating. Care always needs to be understood relationally and contextually. Care, or often a lack of care or care-less space is evident in media representations, education mothering, and intimacy, as I show herein.

Herring's (2013) approach suits a care ethics model of disability, in the context of my three spheres of caring, not least because unconditional love does not always come into the caring story. As he says, 'respect and acceptance of responsibility' are central (Herring, 2013: 25), and it does not necessarily 'require love or even affection. The exhausted disinterested nappy change is caring, even if they don't exactly have that warm fuzzy feel at the time!' (Herring, 2013: 25). This is certainly the case for some mothers or fathers, friends, and education professionals within the context of intellectual disability and caring. It is clear that relationships can be open to abuse, and not without power inequalities, but Herring is attempting to map out legal and social responses to caring relationships, and accepts that not all are the same nor reducible to a 'single set of principles' (Herring, 2013: 26). Actually he suggests that we are all 'ignorant, vulnerable, interdependent individuals, whose strength and reality is not our autonomy, but our relationships with others' (Herring, 2013: 46). He does not, therefore, premise a legal and ethical toolbox on the basis of individual rights, just as I do not propose a care ethics model of disability based on individual rights. As it is, the law labels different groups of people as vulnerable and/or lacking physical or mental capacity, so children, the elderly and disabled people, for example, are deemed in need of protection under the umbrella of the law, but Herring (2013) believes this conceals the vulnerability in us all. There are a number of 'special concessions' made (that is, concessions made because people might be vulnerable and need protecting) when studying for a law degree when it comes to mental health, child law, carer law, elder law and so on, but Herring (2013: 52) would eradicate the special concessions, as they would become the norm. Caring would become the norm.

I am not a legal analyst, and as such realise this is not a legal critique, but more of a means to understand how a care ethics model of disability could work with legal and policy discourses. In addition, I cannot do justice to this in totality, but it is more of a starting point. I will say, significantly, one of the spheres of caring work in the care ethics model of disability is the emotional sphere, and emotions are more often than not left out of the criminal justice system and law textbooks. Yet, despite the fact that caring work is not necessarily about love, 'emotions are central to good care' (Herring, 2013: 57). The exclusion of emotions from the legal process, including love, anger, disappointment and grief, does mean that there is no legal representation in caring work. I can appreciate this when mothers and fathers appeal against a decision, for example, based on the schooling for their intellectually disabled child. From my research, the unemotional father (in this case, the 'unattached' stepfather) speaking at an appeal hearing about his stepson made more headway in getting his point across to those with power on the panel. His wife, the 'emotionally attached' mother defending her position, and her son can cause all kinds of messiness in the meeting room and even be asked to leave in order to gather herself (Rogers, 2007a). This is no longer acceptable if we are to inculcate caring work, care-fullness and ethics into a just society, all within a care ethics model of disability. Therefore, within this, I promote caring relationships, rather than solely carers.

Concluding remarks

Understanding caring relations via the emotional, practical and socio-political spheres will aid a broader understanding of intellectual disability and what it is to be a human being by clarifying knowledge production and understanding how the socio-political, as well as the practical and emotional, merge and facilitate one another. Of course, however, there are some potential dangers lurking in an ethics of care model of disability, just as there are in an ethics of care more generally, if the ideas and practices are misused. After all, if care ethics is about the relational, it can be argued that individuals become vulnerable to a lack of individual identity when considered within this framework. Herring (2013: 179) picks up on Roseneil's (2004) work in identifying this danger, as if we only inhabit a relational self then have we lost the ability to act autonomously, to be separate and to embody individuality? I do not suggest that social justice should move out of the picture, and that we should purely understand human beings as having a psycho-social self. Yet I propose that autonomy is relational. I also come back to Plummer's (2015: 189) pluralistic way of understanding human society where we need a 'down-to-earth everyday loving pragmatism of empathy, fairness, kindness and care. These, indeed, are the little-grounded utopian processes of hope'. I appreciate this way of understanding theory and practice can be difficult, especially for those working within a pure rights-based framework, but individual human rights do not enable us to see the whole picture within relationships, if, for example, exploitation, abuse or violence, systemic or otherwise, are in play. In the next chapter, I identify education and intellectual disability as a case to understand a care ethics model of disability. It is here I begin a process to re-humanise education.

Notes

1   In the context of this book, clearly, there is a huge amount to say about employment and relationships to production when it comes to disability and employment/ unemployment, but this is not covered in this text. However, a care ethics model of disability could be utilised in this area too.
2   A part of this section is reproduced and developed from Philip, Rogers, and Weller (2013: 4–7), I therefore want to thank both Georgia Philip and Susie Weller.
3   In Northern Europe and the UK particularly, there has been a consistent empirical, sociological and feminist engagement with care and caring, with writers such as Graham (1983) and Ve (1989) being important early examples.
4   I take a closer look at *Affiliation, Play*, and *Control over one's environment* in the following chapter, as these capabilities suggest, at the very least, that education and relationships are a medium to spending time with peers and enjoying life, and enable the opportunity to contribute to or control material and political conditions for themselves (or I would suggest interdependency).

5 The Human Development Index was created by Sen, but the reason Nussbaum uses the term *Capabilities* Approach is largely due to the fact that she also recognises non-human animals ought to live a life without abuse and a lack of dignity.

6 This new paradigm 'has had increasing impact on international agencies discussing welfare, from the World Bank to the United Nations Development Programme (UNDP). Through the influence of the Human Development Reports published each year since 1990 by the United Nations Human Development Report Office, it also now affects most contemporary nations, which have been inspired to produce their own capability-based studies of the well-being of different regions and groups in their own societies' (Nussbaum, 2011: x).

7 Most sociological research attempts to make sense of the social and political world by drawing on different human narratives.

8 Of course mutual advantage is problematic. If we take for example the world at large, why would wealthy nations invest in poorer, needy nations (Nussbaum, 2006: 20)? This is evident at a local level when people 'look away' and deny those who are in need of support.

9 Not a social contractarian.

3 Re-humanising education

Introduction

A care ethics model of disability is a global proposition for all areas of social life, but it is within the school system that ethical and care-full work via the emotional, practical and socio-political caring spheres is needed as a starting point. Therefore, it makes sense to examine education and schooling, largely because when it comes to learning, formal or informal, I can identify excessive care-less spaces. Furthermore, the school, as an institution, is a micro social system within the socio-political sphere, where a broader picture of social justice/injustice, exclusion/inclusion, success/failure, and privilege/discrimination can be charted. Education is hugely influential in young people's lives. Therefore, I argue schools must be socially inclusive in the broadest interpretation and enable everyone to engage in a meaningful and care-full education; this is humane. But for intellectually disabled children and young people, this has never been as difficult as it is within the current restrictive and prescriptive curriculum, particularly in the global North (see Cigman, 2007; Rose, 2010; Slee, 2011).[1] Moreover, as I understand from my own schooling experience as a spirited young working class girl, seeing my intellectually disabled daughter struggle through a highly competitive education market, and reading early education philosophers such as Montessori (Standing, 1998) and Pestalozzi (De Guimps, 2004), children learn from doing, creating and discovery (see Smyth, Down and McInerney, 2010). Education should not necessarily be linked to tests *per se*, and as Pestalozzi said in the nineteenth century: 'time for learning is not the time for judgement and criticism' (De Guimps, 2004: 241). All this considered, education is in need of re-humanising.

As it is, Roger Slee (2011) has suggested that we re-frame, re-right, re-search and re-visit all aspects of 'inclusive' education, stating that this is a global political project whereby schooling ought to provide an education in democracy, and further argues that we should disband Ofsted (Office for Standards in Education, Children's Services and Skills) and reconsider league tables. Furthermore, John Smyth and his colleagues, based on their ethnographic study, ask if it is possible to reform schools in order to make them a 'more humane and engaging' space (Smyth, Down and McInerney, 2010: 1997). Without throwing everything up in the air, it seems difficult to envisage how to move forward and re-humanise education without a radical change. Mapping a care ethics model of disability onto the education system, where relational, ethical caring practices are charted via all caring spheres, will benefit *everyone*, not just intellectually disabled people and their families/carers. Importantly, similar to Smyth, Down and McInerney (2010), Slee (2011) questions whether we are actually capable of dismantling exclusion and any practices that feed it. I wonder this too, as exclusionary tactics and care-less spaces are so deeply embedded, implicitly and explicitly (Gillies, 2012; Gillies and Robinson, 2013; Sundaram and Wilde, 2012). No lone person can change this intensely bureaucratic, prescriptive education system, but many are now calling for reformative and radical proposals – a need for creativity, ethical care and social justice in education (Allan, 2010a, 2010b; Luff, 2013; Walker and Unterhalter, 2007). Children, young people, their families, politicians, policymakers, education professionals and support workers are all involved in processes of educating all children, and therefore it is just that a care-full education is promoted.

Currently there are many obstacles and persistent exclusionary tactics with education and schooling. Families, pupils, teachers, professional development strategies, teaching and learning schemes, policy directives and support in the classroom are just a few areas that point towards such barriers and problems (Rose, 2010). Indeed, across all caring spheres struggles with difficult differences require a great deal of caring work from all. It is easier to ignore, deny, and look away from aspects of education and schooling, especially those that seemingly do not involve the wider public. Intellectually disabled people, after all, are not huge contributors to the economic growth of any country, but then I would argue that contributing to the economy does not in essence make a person human. Moreover, this is not the premise of education I would like to promote, nor is it socially and ethically just or caring. Simply to say education is the pathway to employment is not nearly nuanced enough and certainly not caring or ethical. As Tomlinson (2013: 12–13) remarks, not all children and young people will be able to enter the workforce, and consideration ought to be given to 'developing an economy which could employ almost all its citizens, including the lower attainers, with more respect and less paternalism or denigration, and also care for those who may not be employable but are still worthy citizens'.

Education is for everyone, whatever form that might take, and this, I would argue, needs to take place in an inclusive and care-full environment. As I say, it is not at all helpful to 'other', look away from, or exclude children and young people with difficult differences, particularly those who are intellectually disabled, and we know from research that too many young people do not see through their educational journey for a whole range of reasons (Tomlinson, 2013). Not least of these are their feelings of disengagement, alienation and exclusion from a meaningful learning process (Smyth, Down and McInerney, 2010). As a result of exclusionary tactics, social, cultural or economic disadvantage, or disability, vast numbers of pupils are not included, have poor educational experiences and are either marginalised or demonised (Gillies and Robinson, 2010, 2013). The past 15 years or so have seen theoretical and empirical work that has added to debates and addressed different ways of thinking about disadvantage and social inclusion, and all seem to be underpinned by a critical discourse that declares education is failing a large sum of children and young people and therefore needs to be radically reconsidered, which is everybody's business (Allan, 2005, 2010; Benjamin, 2002; Slee, 2011).

Re-humanising education: beyond the call of duty

How can a humanised and caring education be envisaged? Crucially, education practitioners ought to be leaders with a vision for meaningful inclusion (Watkins and Meijer, 2010) as it is the teachers who facilitate learning. Yet it seems teachers are not the leaders and are co-existing alongside students within care-less spaces, although they do find pockets of caring work, and care-full spaces. Smyth, Down and McInerney (2010: 174) found in their research that teachers have some agency in their practice, as they describe a teacher saying 'if I can do something to make it better for kids, I will [...] I haven't hung myself yet so I must be surviving'. This indicates the level of caring and care-full work at a practical and emotional level, but also in terms of the socio-political.

Consider the context of exclusionary practices where a number of children are removed from mainstream education provision and transferred into satellite facilities such as pupil referral units (PRU). These children often have additional and challenging behaviours as well as some difficulties in learning. Pathologising them does not aid a caring process, in fact it harbours carelessness and feeds injustice; nevertheless we are still in this climate. We can see individualistic and therapeutic models in Val Gillies' (2012: 34) ethnographic research, where problems are located within the family or pupil and 'exclusion becomes reinterpreted as a mental state, while inclusion is viewed as a corrective process targeting psychological obstacles to participation' (see also Rogers, 2007a). Gillies goes on to say that currently,

> [s]ocial and relational contexts, power dynamics and the practices and responsibilities of schools are commonly overlooked for a focus on the individual psyche of the troublesome pupil. Attention and resources are directed towards personal change, while the backdrop of socially embedded disadvantage, discrimination, violence and institutional racism are ignored.
>
> (Gillies 2012: 34)

A care ethics model of disability by reconceptualising what education looks like would help to reorganise and reform caring spaces, as a way of challenging the individualistic model, in a way that the social model of disability does not. A care ethics model does not see intellectual capacity as deficit, and neither ought educational processes. Yet inclusion alone, without the care-full and caring work necessary across all spheres, will not work.

It is clear that a reformative change can influence all three spheres of caring work, care-fully for children, caring others, and education professionals. After all, as in Gillies' (2012, forthcoming), Smyth, Down and McInerney's (2010), and Slee's (2010) research, teachers are at the frontline and need caring relations too. My research confirms this position, as I have seen the practical, emotional and socio-political spheres identify such work. For example, Faye, a senior teacher I recently interviewed, who has worked in both mainstream secondary school and for the past eight years in a pupil referral unit (PRU), located in an urban, economically deprived area, emphatically confirms the sentiment from Smyth, Down and McInerney's (2010) research; that of survival. As she told me,

> You live every day, and you never really know what's going to happen. It might be education, but it might be mopping up repercussions around the latest local knife crime where one of our students was involved. I wish I could tell you these are extreme events. My life is one big stress ball.

As the interview progressed it became clear that, although committed to her pupils, the utter exhaustion compels her to continuously look for other work, a job in a less demanding environment. Yet, all good intentions aside, she struggles to let go of her role, due to the nature of the emotional and caring investment, as well as her ethical commitment to the often vulnerable, nevertheless difficult children she deals with on a day-to-day basis.

In addition to the emotional and practical caring work involved, it seems the teachers who do want to rail against the rigid, teaching to test, regulatory directives do have to survive rather than live. This is clearly a socio-political issue where, as I have identified, social intolerance and aversion to difficult differences are played out, and it is care-less and chaotic for all concerned. Policy and political narratives are fragmented around inclusion, which compounds 'confusion, chaos, and considerable damage in the shape of inequality. Race/ethnicity, gender and disability are all addressed in different ways, by different government departments, with different *solutions*' (Allan, 2010a: 28, emphasis in original). In some cases education professionals are silenced, and at worst persecuted and excluded from their employment, for being on the side of those difficult-to-teach others (see Gillies and Robinson, 2010, 2013; Slee, 2011). Education, however, cannot survive on simply 'heroic teachers', but needs radical reform for both schools and communities (Smyth, Down and McInerney, 2010: 187). Ultimately, meaningful, care-full policies are needed, as are caring and just legal procedures (Herring, 2013), and all should develop working relationships with the community *and* in partnership with parents (Hodge and Runswick-Cole, 2008; Rogers, 2011).

As it currently stands, families, teachers, and caring others are often pitched against each other with blame accounting for many narratives I have seen, and this is simply care-less. However, it will take more than a policy directive to address the de-humanising education system which is in place. Caring leadership and vision are vital, and progression towards a care-full education *and community* is a process. But, crucially, all of this will become more consequential within a care ethics model of disability – where socio-political systems are set up within this relational position, and then ethical caring work feeds into emotional and practical experiences. The eradication of social intolerance and aversion to difficult differences is central here. Significantly, when it comes to thinking about teachers' education delivery, student teachers have been asked by researchers about what it is to be 'human and how human differences are socially constructed' (Florian and Rouse, 2010: 193). Florian and Rouse found that many trainee teachers have 'deeply embedded assumptions about human differences that are largely unacknowledged' (Florian and Rouse, 2010: 193). Therefore it is crucial that when doing and planning inclusion and education practice, for example, teachers already believe in the broader socially just and caring approach to teaching differences (Allan, 2003). This includes a meaningful and care-full education and training process, as teachers who are able to successfully include intellectually disabled students constantly have to make decisions about what can be adapted, and teachers need to genuinely believe they can do it (Deng, 2010; Smyth, Down and McInerney, 2010).

However, not only do we need to deal with teachers and families who are pitched against each other; current care-less education exists against a backdrop of vehement anti-inclusion discourse from teachers' unions, policymakers as well as teachers themselves. For example, Douglas Mackie at the Educational Institute of Scotland Presidential Address said in 2004, 'schools must be given the ability to exclude the disruptive'. Indeed, a statement from the National Association of Schoolmasters Union of Women Teachers in the UK claimed '[t]otal inclusion is a form of child abuse, especially if the child is in the completely wrong environment' (Allan, 2010a: 1). I might agree with this, if it was unfeasible to lay to rest the prescriptive education of the current system, but that is not what many are now suggesting; and my proposal is for radical change. Notably, Smyth, Down and McInerney (2010) suggest that neoliberal and neoconservative discourses have worn away young people's experiences by neglecting the meaning-making of the self and identity, and via the exclusion of student's real lives from education. The restricted curriculum, test scores and accountability of teachers restrict this link with their actual lived realities. Therefore it has been suggested that there must be a process of re-writing *and* re-righting identity into education via a humanising pedagogy. It seems unsurprising that pupils want fun, respect and relationships. The socio-political sphere, via policy documents and directives ought to be caring with, about and for children and young people in their learning, and yet they omit fun, curiosity, kindness and compassion.

Thinking about the actual education available to intellectually disabled young people, teaching to test, restricted curriculum and the tensions between an examination culture and inclusive education are contrary to a caring and meaningful education, and we are left with a care-less failing education. Slee's (2011) research narratives seem to be driven by humanity, civility, waste, governance, justice, inclusion and exclusion. Drawing on those known for writing about these broad issues, such as Zygmunt Bauman, Basil Bernstein, Michel Foucault, Martha Nussbaum, and Richard Sennett, he tells a story about 'collective indifference'. Slee (2011) sets the scene where there are many hidden (and not so hidden) exclusionary tactics going on in education globally. For example, the current political state of inclusion contradicts the testing and examination culture (Allan, 2010a; Rogers, 2007a): 'The rhetoric is of educational excellence' (Slee, 2011: 6). Importantly, the concept of 'failure' is talked about metaphorically using the medical term 'triage', thereby suggesting that those 'likely to pull through' will get more attention than those likely to 'die' (or in the case of education, fail their examinations). These narratives around excellence are also played out in Benjamin's (2002) research, where she talks about students who were borderline 'C' grade at GCSE, who would gain more attention from the teachers than those borderline D or E due to their potential to attain that 'C' grade (the hidden pass mark in schools in England and Wales) and raise a school's league table position. This 'teaching to test' and league tabling of school performance is evidently problematic and de-humanising for pupils, parents, education professionals, and additional support staff alike. A re-humanised education would be care-full and creative, for students and education professionals.

Policy and practice rhetoric: stories from the 'inside'

Education is currently interpreted in different ways, and not at all in a way that is helpful or meaningful for intellectually disabled children. Within the practical and socio-political sphere, policymakers could be accused of being on the outside when it comes to identifying what is going on in schools, yet they hold much of the power. Policy 'speak' and rhetoric emerged clearly in an interview I carried out with a senior civil servant in the then UK Department for Education and Skills (DfES).[2] I asked him about what exactly was going on for children identified with 'special educational needs' and their education. He responded by telling me,

> I'm quite clear that there's a lot more to do but I don't think the government, and I can be too apologetic for focusing on results where there is sufficient evidence to suggest that we don't have enough of our children reaching their potential. This isn't an issue of children with learning potential, but we have children whose attainment is clearly below and that means improving the school system. [...] There is a reconciliation and I'm not picking an argument, I think attainment is everything and I think at the same time, mmm, attainment isn't automatically 5 A* to C (GCSEs)[3] but it could be 10 A* to C, equally it could be 10 at D could be

an achievement. I think that attainment is important and if at the end of Key Stage 4[4], erm... teachers could say we really have pushed every one of these children on and they've all achieved something of excellence.

And that's actually the reason why the government has invested in baseline assessments in all the key stages so you can see how the child is doing.

In the very same interview he had already said to me,

> We shouldn't be writing children off based on the fact that they can't get 5 A* to C but need to think more broadly about the areas where they can get [pause]. We have to value the children for where they are no matter what they achieve: the 10% of children who do not reach level 4 at Key Stage 2 or the significant number of children who won't get 5 A* to C at GCSE [...] The ultimate goal that this government has is that we will create a measure of schools value added, to the extent which they help the child move from the level of knowledge that they come into school with and to where they get out, and that hopefully will take a bit of the heat off the league tables which have had an adverse effect but we're talking about children who are always going to be regarded as below what is regarded as age related.

I vividly recall walking away from this interview feeling utterly despondent. I was pleased with myself that I had managed to gain access to a senior official in government. Naïve though too, as I assumed he would open up to me, but the narrative I gained from this interview did not deviate too far from policy directives.

As it is, research suggests that we are writing off a huge number of children, and not just those with intellectual impairments (Gillies, 2012; Slee, 2011; Smyth, Down and McInerney, 2010; Tomlinson, 2013). This explicitly suggests that the narratives gained from my research and those in policy documents are simply rhetoric, basically there as part of the neo-liberal discourse on academic achievement (or perish if intellectually impaired). On reflection, there is probably more to gain from the narrative above than I might have originally thought. What is absolutely clear is that the assessment of children from a young age is about how they achieve, both in relation to summative learning goals (for example, numeracy and literacy targets) and in terms of success relative to their peers both locally and nationally (see Benjamin, 2002). We see this in the tabling of school performance; this is not news. But what is evident is that if education remains so heavily weighted towards particular ways of doing and performing in examinations, lacking creative thought and innovative ways of knowing, then intellectually disabled children, especially those who are unable to read and write, have limited communication and so on, will not be a part of this education experience in any meaningful and caring way, ever. This is inhumane.

I have argued elsewhere that many intellectually disabled children are excluded practically, intellectually and emotionally within mainstream schools (Rogers, 2007a), despite being included on the school roll, and I would add that this is care-less and inhumane. We simply see here the desire to fit everyone into a particular mould and to squeeze them into a very narrow definition of success and achievement. Achievement for any child is about where they are at the time and then where they want to go, with the caring support of those around them. In an interview with Jo, a senior teacher (who was also the designated inclusion officer) working in a mainstream urban school, it is clear that targets are only ever important if relevant. She told me,

> I had a little girl who came into year 7 (aged 12) who was illiterate and innumerate [pause] possibly epileptic, lots of this at the door, can't get her in the door, can't get her out the door, blah, blah came in year 7. Our target for her was that we wanted her to be able to read when she left the school. And her achievement was she went to the front office and read a Wellington Square which is like reading age of 6 type book to the head teacher's secretary. And she sat there as proud as punch that she read this book. To me if the targets that you set are not around, [pause] what the government want [...] you must make sure the kids get the recognition that they deserve and that they can achieve. Another thing was sending her round the shop for cooking ingredients and she came back with the ingredients and the change, on her own at 15. Where does that score on SATs?!![5] Well it don't.

Undoubtedly children have different goals and different learning needs, and what this student might have as a goal when she leaves school is very different from the next child. Thinking about how we understand a caring and care-full education involves a need to move beyond any scores that are noted, and training for teachers must reflect this. Moreover, it seems that, despite the fact that Michael Gove (British politician for the Conservative party) has suggested teachers ought to work longer days and have shorter holidays (Adams and Shepherd, 2013) teachers already spend far too much time on bureaucracy and actually fewer hours in the classroom, according to the OECD (Organisation for Economic Development and Cooperation) (Adams and Shepherd, 2014).

Thus, this socio-political sphere currently maintains little respect and caring for the role of teachers or for a meaningful learning process for children and young people. At the extreme end of the teaching spectrum we have teachers who not only have to manage educational achievements based on national targets that will never be achievable for many intellectually disabled children, but for some of those children, difficult and challenging behaviour can also manifest (Benjamin, 2002; Gillies, 2012; Gillies and Robinson, 2013) thwarting meaningful learning. Jo (the mainstream teacher and 'inclusion' officer) further told me about another 12-year-old student who characterises this 'management' of pupils in addition to teaching the curriculum and all within an 'inclusive' environment as evidence here.

> I've got a girl (Tilly) in year 7 (aged 12) who is [pause] very aggressive, gets involved in a lot of trouble and there was a big fight after school last night, and it came across on the radio [two-way radio transmitter] 'any radio holders there's a fight out the front can any staff get round there', so I've gone running round there with assistant head of year 8, [...] I called Tilly back and she came back and I said 'look Tilly we aint chasing you lot round the borough' and I said 'what's going on?', and she said 'nothing's going on'. I said 'well something's going on, do you want to tell me what's going on', now the girls had come back and she's talking to me and then the head of year arrives 'Oh it's you again is it?' Do you know what I mean! 'Get back to my office I'll deal with you', he shouted, and I thought hang on, you don't even know if Tilly's done anything yet, so off she was marched and I crossed over the road and thought I'd smack that woman in the fucking mouth before long. I thought, you know, how are you going to turn a kid around unless you treat them with some respect, and alright maybe she was the main instigator, but well done for coming over when I called you and that would have been a perfect opportunity and in bowls this head of year, blah, blah, fucking get on with it. And that's what happens all the time.

This type of pastoral and indeed caring and care-full role is obvious, and clearly demanding where teachers are heavily emotionally and practically involved with students, over and above the official curriculum. We saw this with Faye in her narrative above, as she told me about her engagement with pastoral and extra-curricular work. This is also evidenced in other research where education professionals get entangled in their care-full role but are then unable to maintain their caring, due to bureaucratic and systemic obstacles (Benjamin, 2002; Gillies and Robinson, 2013; Slee, 2011). Their ways of being and caring are not simply about whether the children they engage with in school can pass a particular test, and this is a critical point to be made. Jo was unable to get to the bottom of the fight such that, despite Tilly being on her radar as the 'inclusion' officer, she ended up in a care-less space.

This is borne out further in Faye's narrative. She spoke candidly to me about her past eight years in a 'behaviour support placement' (or PRU) and said of behaviour support, 'well it is provision for those pupils who have been excluded from mainstream'. It came to light that some of her students are clearly struggling due to trials that manifest as a result of an extremely challenging home life. She said other pupils have a range of difficulties that are noticeable due to an intellectual impairment as well as being on the autistic spectrum, for example. She revealed to me that her role often involves going to pupils' homes, getting involved with the family and dealing on a day-to-day basis with aggressive and abusive behaviour, and said,

Sometimes you just can't sleep at the end of the day. But you really get embroiled in these lads' lives. Actually the targets for these kids are more often than not to gain a place within further education, often without any GCSEs, or even secure a job if we're really lucky, but I'm trying to get them to turn up to job interviews, tell them how to dress appropriately, not swear and generally coach them. Teaching them? Not sure what that's about anymore!

Importantly, therefore, a 'learning' target for these children is to be able to communicate in a manner that will not marginalise or exclude them from contributing to social life. In reality, it can sometimes be about keeping them from entering the criminal justice system. This must be addressed within the socio-political sphere, not only where policy and systemic changes are made but where all others understand caring as a fundamental part of being human and of social life at a psycho-social level. Not only do trainee teachers need to hear this, but everyone. As it is we know, for example, that young people who are excluded from school often end up in the criminal justice system (Gillies and Robinson, 2013; Rose, 2010; Slee, 2011). Furthermore, research carried out decades ago talks about difficult children, and that a 'web of legal powers, social agencies and practices of judgement and normalisation began to spread around troubled and troublesome children' (Rose, 1989: 131) (see also Donzelot, 1979). Yet we still see the medicalisation of difficult behaviour suggesting the naughty, fidgety, disengaged child is maladjusted, troubled, disordered and genetically compromised and can be 'fixed', treated, eliminated or at least managed out of sight. The policymakers, and indeed politicians, do not want these hard to teach and reach children disrupting the manageable flow of education, largely because these children blemish the national academic targets.

There are extremes here where young people are unable to communicate verbally, read and write, or behave in socially acceptable ways, but this is how it is. Significantly, there are some difficulties we can address where we have to work in a care-full manner with particular behaviour issues, but there are also children who will never be able to read beyond a very basic level, if at all, particularly those with severe and profound intellectual impairments. Certainly, I feel confident in saying that if we take out regimented prescriptive testing then we might actually be able to begin to have a caring, care-full, ethical and socially just education system for all. This will, I imagine, not be popular with everyone, but there is evidence to suggest that '*what is good for pupils with SEN is good for all pupils* in inclusive settings. Good teaching approaches benefit all pupils' (Watkins and Meijer, 2010: 242, emphasis in original). In addition, there are national and international government directives as well as legal obligations to educate and care for all children and young people. For example, in the UK, 'Every Child Matters' (ECM, 2004) promotes a meaningful sense of well-being for all children and claims to foster radical improvements. 'Education for All' (UNESCO) is positioned as a global, broadly defined inclusive education strategy, and the Individuals with Disabilities Education

Act (IDEA) in the USA has influenced the levels of opportunities for disabled students. These are just a few of the policy contexts within which education is addressed as a means to promote inclusion and appropriate learning internationally. However, this is not currently working for all, and therefore these policies and directives are arguably meaningless.

In the research identified here there is call for creativity. Yet within the confines of Michael Gove's interpretation of creativity, it is nigh on impossible to actually be creative without first learning musical scales, mathematics, writing skills and so on, depending on what skill you want to develop (Robinson, 2013). This is yet further rhetoric around what creativity, education and learning are about. For example, I learned how to play the recorder without reading notes, I taught myself basic guitar by looking at pictures, and I learned how to perform on stage before studying Stanislavski or Brecht. I do not have an intellectual impairment, but the point is that creativity, genuine creativity, can be messy and disruptive, but more importantly, no one really learns to create without motivation, and you cannot enforce motivation. 'The real driver of creativity is an appetite for discovery and a passion for the work itself. When students are motivated to learn, they naturally acquire the skills they need to get the work done' (Robinson, 2013: n.p.). To make a point, my intellectually disabled daughter tends to learn skills that are totally embroiled in motivation and desire, for example, a desire to communicate with others and play games, so she has learned how to use the iPad. A wish to give gifts means she learns how to make bracelets out of coloured bands. The other end of the intellectual spectrum is no different, when it comes to creative thinking. For example, when I ask a student of mine to think creatively, theoretically, innovatively, it can be a struggle as they have progressed through a system that does not privilege this, but teaches students to learn facts and recall from memory via rote learning. Yet I have on occasion a student who will gain an extremely high grade despite some 'flaws' in their composition because of their understanding of a concept, or their innovative interpretation of an issue, largely because they are passionate about the subject matter. Critically, students do want to be involved and we need to think about hearing (and doing something about) all voices in the mix, not least of all pupils (Allan, 1999a; Benjamin, 2002; Gillies and Robinson, 2010, 2013; Jones and Gillies, 2010; Lawson, 2010; Smyth, Down and McInerney, 2010).

Shelvin (2010), for example, explains that the children in his research about disability and education wanted to talk about access, ambition and achievement and then voice their concerns. Participation for all is crucial, and indeed ethical (Rogers and Ludhra, 2012; Rogers with Tuckwell, in press), but must not be carried out tokenistically (Gillies and Robinson, 2010). Unsurprisingly, children want to be included when adults are making decisions about their lives and their futures. Moreover, they want to be prepared for adult life, as Shelvin (2010) found in his research, and this ought to be a possibility whether a child is dependent, independent or interdependent. In truth, the students in Shelvin's (2010) research saw education as a crucial place to learn not only about the formal curriculum, but about social, cultural and personal issues too. This aspect of 'hearing' about children and young people's experiences is essential in understanding the particular positions from which education is experienced. Moreover, when it comes to hearing what politicians, policy-makers, teachers and pupils have to say, their narratives are indeed important, but so are appeals from academic researchers. Allan (2005), Slee (2011), and Smyth, Down and McInerney (2010), for example, are calling in different ways for a more creative and encouraging space for children and young people to learn in. The demand for care, creativity and trust, where educational leadership is inspirational and the student voice is heard, is vital. With regard to social inclusion, which I would suggest is the key motivator in thinking about ethics, caring and a re-humanised education for intellectually disabled people, we could argue for an ethical inclusion project (Allan, 2005). Nussbaum writes of

> a society that acknowledges its own humanity, and neither hides us from it nor it from us; a society of citizens who admit that they are needy and vulnerable, and who discard the grandiose demands for omnipotence and completeness that have been at the heart of so much misery and human misery, both public and private.
>
> (Nussbaum 2004: 17)

Significantly, what some of the authors above address in particular, either implicitly or explicitly, is humanity, human differences or being human in one way or another, in relation to the education of children and young people, their parents, educators and carers, and yet many people continue to look away from or deny difficult differences.

Looking away (Othering) is de-humanising

The damning media attention 'difficult' young people gain, and the over-governed, over-surveyed and over-assessed education system young people inhabit, which in turn allows for league tabling and competitive schooling, is evident. We can see this too in a global context (Allan, 1999a; Rogers, 2007a; Rose, 2010; Smith, Down and McInerney, 2010). In their study, Smyth and his colleagues alert the reader to a managerialist and consumer driven society that has had a negative impact upon the education process. They found students were like clients to be filled with knowledge that resulted in certificates, making them marketable. This is de-humanising. But for intellectually disabled students where their 'market value' is below any meaning and they are fit to be discarded in terms of human worth, it is magnified. Teachers, within their prescribed local and national directives, deliver a restricted and restricting curriculum to test, disabling creativity and hindering spontaneity. All of these things increase the divide between those who are disadvantaged and disabled and those who are not. Smyth, Down and McInerney's (2010) focus is on 'doing', so, for example, doing schooling, doing identity, doing policy, which is a position that enables and promotes social justice, beginning with young people and their social and cultural spaces. The principle is that education ought to be the driving force behind young people making sense of their lives and identities, leading them to contribute to creating a socially just and democratic society. Ultimately, Smyth, Down and McInerney (2010) suggest there is a poverty of opportunity amongst learners, and this is played out across schools, feeding disadvantage and narratives of toxicity. These findings are particularly poignant, therefore, in an attempt to re-humanise education, yet currently intellectually disabled people are not positioned as change makers in any way.

Important too in Smyth, Down and McInerney's (2010) research, for me here in discussing intellectual disability and being human, is identity formation, largely because they unpick 'doing identity formation' in relation to meaning-making. Crucially, the consumption of dominant social images and experiences makes the young people who they are and influences how they shape themselves, in the context of family and school life. With reference to Adorno and Horkheimer and 'the culture industry', Smyth, Down and McInerney (2010) draw out aspects of the visual, particularly media-produced images, branding and everyday material life. So, for example, the clothes one wears and the gadgets one buys feed into how social status develops and identity is formed. This aspect of children being caught in a 'materialistic trap' has been aired in the UK news as a result of a Unicef report (Ramesh 2011) suggesting that a meaning-making process goes on within and beyond school which associates material goods with happiness. This feeds into the de-humanising and care-less education available to intellectually disabled young people, as many do not have the intellectual capacity, communication skills, or social maturity to enter into this consumer game-playing. That is not to say many do not desire it; just as many young people produce and consume images, including large sporting events, pop concerts, eroticism and video and computer games. In fact it seems this consumerism is the drug of the masses and, as they quote from Adorno and Horkheimer, '[p]leasure always means not to think about anything, to forget suffering even where it is shown' (Smyth, Down and McInerney, 2010: 114).

There are three things going on here: one, intellectually disabled young people might struggle with (or indeed ignore) consumer pressures; two, it is often happening within a formal or informal education setting; and three, all this consumption by other young people enables children and adults alike to look away from suffering, exclusion and dehumanising care-less processes. This turning away from suffering, or rather being seduced by goods, can lead to denial of abhorrent things going on elsewhere (Cohen, 2001) or invoke a 'collective indifference' (Slee, 2011) which is crucial for understanding the socio-political sphere in the context of a care ethics model of disability. Indeed, anyone who does not have an impairment can feel good about themselves not only by buying into mass consumer culture, but also by fetishising guilt

(Cremin, 2012). As I have already identified in Chapter 1, this happens via a global conscience when people enter into a charitable relationship with disability stories at mass telethons such as Children in Need and Comic Relief. Therefore it might be that we can behave in a particular way (ignore the intellectually disabled person in school) if we raise some money for the poor tragic cases on the television.

Regarding other tactics used to exclude and position people as 'other', Slee (2011) discusses the parallel between education and health, for example, suggesting that the masking of pain with drugs can alleviate or dull the everyday 'pain', be that depression with Prozac or behavioural problems with Ritalin, used in many cases due to a diagnosis around Attention Deficit Hyperactivity Disorder (ADHD). I am not suggesting the drugs do not work, and recognise that this point is controversial and provocative, as we do not have to go too far to see that in late modern society, especially in the global North, we have become used to eliminating the 'pain' of everyday life, whether through drugs or 'talking cures' (Craib, 1994). But this *is* provocative, especially in talking to teachers and parents who experience day-to-day difficulties within care-less spaces. Do you tell a mother at the end of her tether that she simply has to deal with life as she contemplates suicide due to everyday difficulties, lack of social care and social exclusion?[6] What do you say to a mother who recently told me that whilst she realises her 15-year-old son probably does not have ADHD, 'if he didn't take the Ritalin he wouldn't learn a thing at school'? However difficult these issues, it is important to recognise the negative and care-less impact of trying to eliminate difficult differences (hiding from them) rather than working with them in a care-full manner (recognising and dealing with these difficult differences). Slee (2011) candidly, in his research, takes the reader through different cultural contexts but soon recognises that once 'home' it is all too easy to drift into a 'collective indifference' – a sense that the disadvantage and poverty is somewhere far away. This 'collective indifference' is somewhat similar to the 'denial' that Stan Cohen (2001) discusses in his thesis, as he talks of how both people and societies deny psychological difficulties or societal atrocities as many avert their gaze from difficult differences.

Slee (2011) suggests that we allow exclusion to take place because in many ways we do not *allow ourselves* to see it, even though we see it all the time via the Internet and rolling global reporting. At a more 'local' level, I have seen this played out (Rogers, 2007a) where a mother with a disabled and 'difficult' child experienced exclusion in the playground as other mothers petitioned the head teacher to exclude her son. This I would consider to be a very care-less space. The mothers with their 'normal' children wanted to be rid of this boy who disrupted both their children's and their lives practically, and indeed emotionally. If these mothers and their 'normal' children do not have to see this difficult and different child they can deny his existence. So a mother experiences exclusion in the playground because her son, who has ADHD, is disruptive to his school peers and their education. Other mothers do not like the disruptive or difficult child, or his mother. They both pose a danger: to their 'normal' children, to the equilibrium of the school and classes, to the teacher and other education professionals, to the delivery of the curriculum, to the playground, to maternal communication. All of these aspects of school life are part of the emotional, practical and socio-political caring spheres. They feed into and out of each other, and intellectual disability, or social and behavioural differences, fractures and disturbs. This all takes place in a context where socio-political narratives via policy directives privilege academic excellence, promote an examination culture and work against caring practices, where those who are not traditionally academically able exist. This in turn impacts upon how, practically and emotionally, we all engage with such everyday occurrences. Therefore, instead of focusing on such 'dangerous' people who underline human vulnerability, lack of reason, and dependency, we all need to establish caring practices within a care ethics model of disability, where interdependence is privileged and caring workers are valued indiscriminately (see Mahon and Robinson, 2011). This could be tricky considering the legal system has such power (Herring, 2013).

Cohen's (2001: 52) work, where '[d]enial and normalization reflect personal and cultural states in which suffering is not acknowledged', works within a broad human rights and sociological frame, and discusses human rights violations and mass atrocities in analysing denial. I build upon this denial as Slee (2011) says that both the everyday looking away from people who experience disadvantage and the rhetoric around inclusion policies and practice feed a 'collective indifference', and, I would argue, care-lessness. Competition and individualism compound a lack of human connection and hence lead to an uncivil society and exclusion. Who is to be included then? Slee asks 'who will be left as the "normal child" once the cartographers of human disorders hang up their tools, dust off their workbench and fold their aprons?' (2011: 41). But as we delve deeper it seems Slee is suggesting that those who are strangers or who are Other are those who many people *fear* are problematic. Importantly, and indeed again openly, Slee (2011: 52) shares with the reader a recollection of childhood memory about how he befriended a disabled and disadvantaged boy and then ignored him at school, also recounting how his mother said (under her breath and as Slee recalls) about a disabled girl who died in a domestic accident, '[i]t's a tragedy, but a blessing'. These types of othering actions by children, and comments about the 'tragedy of disability' are not unusual, and, as Slee puts it, the sentiments that leak into the social psyche are that disabled people are '[b]etter off dead than disabled according to this calculus of human value' (Slee, 2011: 52). This human calculus is worthy of further thought as Jock Young (1999) talks of human worth by discussing credit ratings. He maps a move from inclusion to exclusion and suggests the mode of exclusion is one that shifts and is also dependent on one's 'credit rating', from the wealthy to the 'dangerousness of the incarcerated'. In my previous work (Rogers, 2007a) I suggested that there is a 'credit rating' for people who are intellectually disabled, only their 'credit' is calculated within a mental ability, aesthetic beauty and 'appropriate' social interaction frame. It is this continuum of 'normality' that renders the child excluded and difficult, with a very low 'credit rating' in terms of 'worth', which leads to their ultimate exclusion.

In thinking, then, about exclusion, othering, human calculus and care-less spaces, inclusive education is not a 'technical problem to be solved through an ensemble of compensatory measures' (Slee, 2011: 108); it is considered far more radical and creative. However, even though integration has been seen as an assimilation process, it was a project of political struggle and cultural change, unlike inclusion, which has thus far seemingly not challenged the dominant culture. Some teachers' unions, policymakers and structures enable 'looking away'. Notably, in Slee's research he tells the reader that he was withdrawn from an expert panel on how to deal with a boy who was causing some problems for the school due to his potential vulnerability and personal circumstances. Slee wanted to find a way to support this family, not a way to exclude the boy, hence his withdrawal by the other panel members, those in control, as this was seen as a much more difficult way forward. It was far easier to exclude the difficult boy and his family. But it is not just Slee, as an 'expert' wheeled into to toe the party line, who is silenced by his dismissal from this official process. For example, Gillies and Robinson (2010, 2013) found that one of the behavioural support unit (their catch-all term for units that house difficult to teach young people) managers, 'after 26 years as a teacher [...] received a redundancy notice in the context of cuts to the school budget' (2013: 50). This could be interpreted as a silencing of the politically active and caring staff member who was outspoken and certainly positioned himself on the side of the students, because 'Dave's passionate determination to secure justice for his pupils did not endear him to his colleagues in the mainstream school' (Gillies and Robinson, 2013: 50). It seems, therefore, that we retreat from difficult differences and continue to sanitise processes in whatever way we can. Nevertheless, how ethical and caring is it to look away, to eliminate from view or to silence? Not caring at all, and is indeed very care-less.

Towards a politics of desire and care-full inclusion: cases to learn from

Martha Nussbaum's (2004, 2006, 2011) and Julie Allan's (1999a, 2003a, 2003b, 2005, 2010a, 2010b) works are pertinent here as their enquiry goes beyond the school in thinking about inclusion as a broader political and ethical project. It is for these reasons I discuss their work in more detail below.

Julie Allan and ethical inclusion

Drawing particularly on Foucault, but also other philosophers of difference, namely Deleuze and Guattari, Julie Allan suggests a move towards ethical inclusion and a politics of desire. Allan has written a great deal on inclusive education, the ethics of inclusion and the sociology of disability, much of which has emphasised difficulties in learning both within and beyond Scotland (UK). Her work began with empirical qualitative research as a doctoral student in mainstream schools in Scotland, analysing narratives of mainstream school pupils, children identified with 'special needs', teachers, other education professionals, and parents (Allan, 1999a). She positioned this research within a Foucauldian framework, and using Foucault's 'box of tools' identified the transgressive behaviour of disabled students and found mainstream pupils generally to be the gatekeepers of inclusion, amongst other things (Allan, 1999a, 1999b). The Foucauldian framework of 'hierarchical surveillance', 'normalising judgements' and 'the examination' allowed the governing of pupils identified with 'special educational needs' (SEN), and inclusive education to be itself under the spotlight, philosophically, politically and practically. This enabled an analysis of official discourses around 'special' education and an understanding of how these discursive networks 'construct the pupils as passive subjects, tied to others through control and constraint and to their self-formed identities' (Allan, 1999a: 3).

Importantly, Foucault's archaeologies, genealogies and ethics have been influential in Allan's research, aiding understanding of inclusive education, particularly with regards to its mechanisms of surveillance and governance (Allan, 1999a). Intellectually disabled children, teachers and parents are all under scrutiny in an attempt to make these difficult others fit in. For example, one of the transparent mechanisms of surveillance is the statement (or record in Scotland) of special needs.[7] This official document identifies and pathologises 'difficult to teach' children's educational, and sometimes pastoral, requirements in an attempt to make them fit within the norms of that context, so in this instance within the school environment and within the context of particular learning and behavioural outcomes. The statement, or record, of educational needs is also a collection of 'expert' comments that often include, for example, teacher, special educational needs co-ordinator, educational psychologist, physiotherapist, and parental views on the child. Or at least that is what is supposed to happen. However, we know that this is not necessarily the case, as some parents want a statement (or record) of 'needs' to enable support (which is ultimately what it is for) while others find the whole process of intense surveillance an exercise in apportioning blame, and one which is extremely care-less.

The following narrative highlights this governance, where a mother in my research (Rogers, 2007a: 77–78) whose son, aged 12, had been diagnosed with ADHD and Asperger syndrome, told me he did not have a statement (at the time of interview) as he was in the process of being assessed. It was the 'school that called in the family consultation unit' assuming that something was 'not quite right' at home. The whole family (mother, father, three children and the au pair) were asked to attend, and I was told it was the only time she had taken her other two children to any meeting related to her disabled son. Their experience of it was short but memorable.

The family consultation unit was an absolute disaster we were slated... as a family. We had lack of continuity of support at home because we had au pairs, and me working, and we had [my husband] who came over dreadfully. He can't handle anything like that. I mean he was gazing at the ceiling and I thought 'shit we're just being hung here'. I was still in my uniform [nurse] because one of my clinics had run late which went down a hoot, and I staggered in with my briefcase and Mark was under the chair and round the room, (my daughter) wouldn't talk at all... it was just before she went on anti-depressants and she resented being there and said 'there's nothing wrong with me'... and he [her oldest son] was laughing manically because Mark was so awful, so (her oldest son) is laughing and thinking 'what the hell are we doing here', and I just winked at him, we're on the same wavelength, and I could see this is bad news and I thought, 'oh well what the hell', and they started on about Mark and 'are his symptoms relieved when his bowels are opened?' [She breaks down laughing]. And [her husband] who's on another planet anyway, has never come across anything psychiatric in his life ever, never, and thought 'what on earth's going on?' He got lost on that and said, 'how does having your bowels open... how does that help us in here?' And he got very agitated... 'to listen to this crap', which didn't go down very well because as far as the professionals were concerned, he [my husband] wasn't open-minded and willing to help and change and move on... we came out of there *us* needing 'intensive family support work', I mean everything. You name it... we had a whole list, I said 'get stuffed! You'll never see me cross your doorstep again'. And so that, according to the professionals, was 'objectionable, un-cooperating.... Blah, blah blah', back to us again, the family. So I went back to the hospital and said, 'if you ever put us through that again you can get stuffed as well... it's an insult that you sent us to a place like that'.

I have detailed this here as it is clear that this whole family were very uncomfortable with being surveyed even though this may have come across, to the 'experts', as them being difficult and uncooperative. I would also suggest that this interaction took place in a care-less space. Within a care ethics model of disability, via the three caring spheres, we can begin to identify the potential for becoming more caring, and care-full.

Revisiting transcripts from my earlier data, there was another similar case where I interviewed mother and father together. This excerpt from a discussion they had about their experience of being 'investigated' again highlights the care-less space that parents exist within when being surveyed:

FATHER: The only side of it was he saw the psychiatrist there, and they gave us the diagnosis there. He wanted to see all of us at the same time, d'you remember? He got all of us in the room at the same time.

MOTHER: You *loved* it didn't you? (Sarcastic)

FATHER: I did. I thought it was absolutely fantastic. (Sarcastic)

MOTHER: You didn't have a very high regard for social workers to start with, do you? (laughs) We thought oh great and we all went in and nothing happened did it? They just asked us a load of stupid questions didn't they?

FATHER: He was weird wasn't he? He asked me if I was all right, and I said 'as far as I know' and he said 'what do you mean?' And I said 'well I haven't been told that I'm not so I assume I am' (Mother is laughing in the background). And he sort of (he laughs) because he was really really strange and then we were trying to drop huge hints that we didn't want to talk about (son) in front of him and (apparently) I was being so obtuse that [...]

MOTHER: [...] Someone might have thought there was something wrong with you (laughing)

FATHER: Either I looked like I was totally barmy or I was trying to get somewhere and in the end (mother) said look we're trying to imply that we don't want to talk in front of him [...] it was funny wasn't it?

MOTHERS: That's another thing that people don't seem to realise that you don't want to say things in front of your child.

These narratives underline the surveillance of children and their families which often happens before a statement (or record) is issued. In cases where intellectual impairment is more significant, whilst the assessment process might be marginally different and happen earlier on in the child's life, most of the time all the family want is a caring and care-full relationship. They certainly do not realise that they might be blamed, or at the very least, feel blamed for their child's difficulties and impairments.

The professionals had an agenda (to find out if there were any problems in the family, and to see if they could support them), and the family, by being viewed as uncooperative, are assigned the label of a 'dysfunctional family' in need of 'intensive family support work'. As it is, parents, and often the mother, stand as mediators between the private world of the family and the public, especially when it comes to education (Crozier and Reay, 2004; Read, 2000; Vincent, 2000) which involves regulation of the child's social, moral and intellectual well-being. It is hardly surprising, therefore, that the impact of being told, or made to feel, that a mother, and indeed family, are not doing the 'job' properly is immense, especially given the emotional angst of what has been (and may still be) going on, as evidenced in the following chapter. Therefore, in thinking about these examples, and in the context of Allan's work, Foucault is considered important to the study of 'special needs' and education theoretically and methodologically, as it seems governance and surveillance of the child, and indeed the family, by the 'expert' (and within the socio-political sphere) feeds into a normalising discourse whereby the difficult to teach child and their family are positioned as other, and therefore in need of remedy (Rogers, 2007a). It seems from the research that I have discussed so far that none of this is carried out in a care-full manner. Trying to mould or reconfigure a child or family that simply does not fit within the cultural norms at any one time, for example, where academic attainment is privileged over creativity, or human flourishing, is ultimately dehumanising.

Studies carried out by Foucault, although not empirical, are seen to be critical in understanding power, governance and surveillance in various aspects of modern cultures, institutions and discourses. Archeologically, his studies of medicine (Foucault, 2003) and madness (Foucault, 1989), for example, provide the reader with a history of 'truths' where human beings are subjected to surveillance. Consequently patients are hospitalised, where their bodies are objectified and mental illness is contained and examined within specialised institutions. The move is away from the domain of the private into a site that is visible and therefore controlled. Both the 'fractured' physical and mental body are spoken about as abnormal, always in relation to a certain norm, such that a process of normalisation evolves. This is important when trying to understand a dehumanised education, as normalisation, according to Jean Carabine (2004), is a process defining appropriate and acceptable behaviour, it operates in a regulatory capacity and works to 'produce differentiating effects and fragmented impacts which are in turn variously regulatory, penalizing or affirmative in respect to different groups' (Carabine, 2004: 38). All of this has an impact on intellectually disabled children and young people, on their learning.

Moreover, Foucault's genealogical work moves the focus on from descriptive accounts via discourses to an analysis of more discursive practices (macro to micro) in search of points of resistance (Allan, 1999b). So prisoners and imprisonment (Foucault, 1991) and sexuality (Foucault 1990) were analysed via techniques of power within institutions such as prisons, where power is considerably more anonymous, functional and individualised. Furthermore, it occurs in relation to, and between, individuals. Thus, 'in a system of discipline, the child is more individualised than the adult, the patient more than the healthy man, the madman and the delinquent more than the normal and the non-delinquent' (Foucault, 1991: 193). Significantly with regards to intellectually disabled people, who are often infantilised based on their mental capacity, 'when one wishes to individualize the healthy, normal, and law-abiding adult, it is always by asking him how much of the child he has in him' (Foucault, 1991: 193). This is always illuminating, as we often manage education objectives based on consideration of a maturity of mind, including the ability to read and write, and to be able to answer particular questions in a particular way. This limits any progress in moving towards a caring and just education.

As a consequence of Foucault's work, as already suggested, he identifies three mechanisms of surveillance: hierarchical observations, normalising judgements and the examination. Hence it is here that Allan (1999a) begins her journey through an analysis of special education and inclusion, as 'these techniques appear to shape many of the experiences of children with special needs and are so sophisticated that "inspection functions ceaselessly. The gaze is alert everywhere"' (Allan, 1999a: 20). Allan identifies that Foucault's work is predominately about discourses, which has its limitations, but identifies that the genealogical work, importantly, does take into account the political and economic concerns of the time. As a result, Allan, as I have identified, using Foucault's 'box of tools' is able to analyse both the official discourses surrounding special educational needs, and those working within schools, classrooms, educational administration and so on. Therefore, we can see that mechanisms or techniques of power are positioned within special education, via Allan's qualitative narratives, discourse analysis and policy interrogation. Consequently, hierarchical observation is noted where children identified with special needs in mainstream schools are kept under surveillance, via the statement (England and Wales) or record (Scotland) of needs. This framework of hierarchical surveillance involves both professionals and parents, but 'within this hierarchy, parents' knowledge of their child was subjugated by that of professionals' (Allan, 1999a: 76). More often than not, the report detailed 'objective statements of fact', such as noted here: '[Raschida] suffers from retinitis pigmentosa and subsequent restricted visual field' (Allan, 1999a: 76), or subjective and negative accounts of parents' involvement, as suggested here in one record of need from a professional's perspective: '[a] major problem could be Brian's parents' acceptance of the need for a special school placement' (Allan, 1999a: 77). Moreover, as Allan points out, Brian's parents were criticised 'for being unreasonable' (Allan, 1999a: 77) and went on to say it was common that parents were described in highly emotive ways. This still occurs today, where parents are blamed for difficult parent/professional relations, as I identified above (Rogers, 2007a, 2011).

These hierarchical observations feed into normalising judgements where certain behaviours are pathologised (for example, obstinacy, unpredictable behaviour and moods), always in relation to abnormal/normal binary positions: 'The normalising judgements of the teachers were based on a gaze which saw certain things and ignored others' (Allan, 1999a: 79). But all aspects of behaviour and learning were judged against what the expected behaviour or level of attainment was for their age. This, in turn, allowed the gaze of 'the examination' to enter. Thus, '[b]efore a multi-disciplinary assessment of a child with special needs takes place, the suspicion of abnormality needs to be voiced' (Allan, 1999a: 22), and this can take place at birth, or later on when a child reaches school and teachers or parents notice inconsistencies in learning, for example. Early childhood providers or the school may then make comparisons based on norms, evidencing abnormality, and, as Allan continues, '[b]y the time the child undergoes a formal assessment, there is usually little doubt as to the existence of an abnormality or special need, although this notion of difference is, of course, socially constructed' (Allan, 1999a: 22). This process is deeply problematic and fractures any caring and care-full education process.

However, not content with unpicking narratives alone in working towards an understanding of the mechanisms of inclusive education, Allan has played key advisor roles in policy committees as an insider/outsider voice, especially in Scottish Parliament (Allan, 2003a), and has in turn critically engaged with this political process as well as excavating theoretical works more recently (Allan, 2005, 2010a). Notably she has certainly not done this to curry favour, as her seemingly unwavering push towards inclusion (with special education as the enemy) has provoked some vitriolic responses, especially from places such as those already noted above, including teachers' unions. The National Association of Schoolmasters Union of Women Teachers in the UK suggested in 2001 that full inclusion was a form of child abuse (Allan, 2010a: 1), and then a more personal attack on Allan was a response from a teacher regarding inclusion,

> 'experts' such as Julie Allan [...] are constantly turning a blind eye to the complaints of teachers that this ideology, great on paper, simply does not work. [...] Surely our human rights are being infringed. [...] The education system will keep functioning without ... Allan. It cannot cope without teachers.
>
> (Allan, 2010a: 153)

All of this came about in the context of Mary Warnock suggesting that maybe she did make a mistake in pursuing integration for *all* children back in the late 1970s, and stating that inclusion is now 'disastrous' (Allan, 2005: 22).

Thus it seems writing on inclusion as a way of thinking about a caring and care-full education is not an easy or straightforward path, but within a politics of inclusion as an ethical project (and I would argue caring), interestingly quoting from David Bowie, Allan implies the only thing to do, 'if you want to contribute to culture, or politics, or music, or whatever, is to utilise your own personae rather than just music. The best way to do this is to diversify and become a nuisance everywhere' (Bowie [1976], cited in Allan, 2010a: 153). To stick with a music theme, I suggest we do as Sinatra sang, and 'do it my way'. Bowie, Sinatra, Allan, and others have suggested that if one wants to make a difference, and indeed contribute meaningfully to debates, the path is not necessarily straightforward, nor indeed a popularity contest. We all need to be in some way provocative, and keep buzzing around the earholes of those with more power, indeed, be a nuisance. Of course this is easier said than done as, when it comes to teachers for example, Allan suggests there are limits to what they 'can be asked to do and they need to feel that they belong to an education system that recognises their valuable contribution to the lives of children and young people and the pressures they face' (Allan, 2010a: 130). However, she goes onto to say that the struggle is highly political.

With this in mind then, Allan has continued to pursue inclusion, but knowing that we need to think differently in making sense of it. Therefore she continues to follow a more philosophical route in attempting to add to political debates and utilises philosophers of difference. For instance, we already know that she engages with Foucault, but she also draws upon Deleuze, Guattari and Derrida in an attempt to re-vision inclusion and inclusive education not as something to attain or a problem to sort out but as a puzzle to pursue in a rhizomic[8], rather than hierarchical, fashion (Allan, 2010a). Moreover, she suggests a reframing of inclusion as an ethical project that begins with the self and moves into a 'politics of desire' (Allan, 2005: 293). The success of this ethical project is largely based on the desire of people to get involved, and it is everybody's business (Slee, 2010), which is why the self as a work in progress, and desire, are critical to this project. I would argue that this goes beyond the self, as within a feminist ethics frame we always exist in relation with an Other. This ethical and caring project needs to include this type of caring and care-full work. Furthermore, in thinking about inclusion, for example, it is not necessarily the desire of everybody, as we have seen, because when 'inclusion is framed as an ethical project that leads to a politics of desire, *special educational needs* becomes identified as "the main danger" (Foucault 1984: 343) to disabled people and as an inappropriate basis for pedagogy' (Allan, 2005: 293, emphasis in original).

There is much research from special educationists, with teachers and those engaging with parental narratives, that suggests inclusion is, at best, inappropriate and, at worst, damaging for all concerned (Allan, 2010a, 2010b). For some of us, however, the politics of inclusion, care, ethics and social justice is worth pursuing beyond the school gates and into a psycho-social sphere where, more often than not, life is messy and sometimes disappointing (Craib, 1994), but never dull.[9] Ultimately, in a project focused on ethics and inclusion, I can think about how we consider being in an inclusive, but more importantly a caring and care-full, society where tolerating difference is simply not good enough, because to 'tolerate difference is to "put up with" rather than accept. To accept difference is not to accept failure and underachievement but to accept the idiosyncratic aspects of the human being within this social context' (Rogers, 2007a: 177). Despite this negativity, Allan does believe that inclusion is still a worthwhile pursuit and can be aided by philosophical concepts, even if this means feeling insecure and uncertain about the transformatory process. She suggests that 'we can never be done with the project of inclusion and must continue to puzzle over it together with those who stand to gain most' (Allan, 2010a: 164). In this context I see that in a volatile political climate, Allan is unwavering in her push towards inclusion as an ethical, and I would argue humane and caring, project. This aids a move towards re-humanising education. Martha Nussbaum, in a different way, is suggesting a broader ethical project based on capabilities, but is equally committed to political change and social justice.

Martha Nussbaum, just education and re-humanising

I have already discussed Martha Nussbaum's work in some detail in Chapter 2, but revisit it here to identify its use with respect to the exclusion of vulnerable children, particularly those with intellectual impairments, as any 'decent society must address their needs for care, education, self-respect, activity, and friendship' (Nussbaum, 2006: 98). A just and caring society would not hinder the development of intellectually disabled people; instead it would support participatory inclusion in all areas of life, including education and, where possible, political life. The ethical caring involved needs to be non-exploitative. Nussbaum (2006), in her thesis on justice, draws on classical theory much of the time, and says that those being 'spoken to' via the social contract, for example, were men. Others, namely women, children and the elderly, were not seen as economically productive and were therefore excluded from this discourse and from full participation in civil society. A great deal of this exclusion in recent history has been resolved *to an extent,* but no 'social contract doctrine, however includes people with severe and atypical physical and mental impairments in the group of those by whom basic political principles are chosen' (Nussbaum, 2006: 15).

We know that historically, in the main, disabled people were excluded and there was no political movement aimed at effecting change. Intellectually disabled people were certainly not included within any meaningful education. Thinking, then, about social justice, and indeed inclusion, therein lays the problem. They are not considered full citizens and they certainly struggle to get their voices heard, and at worst are de-humanised. As it is, powerful others make decisions about people's capacity to participate in civil life based on such things as cognitive ability, reason and rationality, and physical strength for example (Nussbaum, 2006: 16). This clearly excludes many intellectually disabled people from contributing to and participating as citizens in social and policy life, and indeed in their education. To this end, institutions, including educational establishments, 'must be sustained by the good will of citizens, but they also embody and teach norms of what a good and reasonable citizen is' (Nussbaum, 2004: 16). If 'good will' is not carried out in a caring manner, or if it is not considered a priority for all, like with the teachers above and their senior colleagues, then a caring and care-full education cannot exist. Namely, a caring, just and re-humanised education will address all three caring spheres where all citizens will employ care-full relations, and this can be applied to intellectual disability, but also to other intersections of society.

I have acknowledged a need for a caring and creative education and curriculum, as Nussbaum emphasises the need for decent living conditions and a creative space. She adds, as I have already said, that this must enable human beings to do and be who they want to be (Nussbaum, 2011), and further asks what 'real opportunities are available?' (Nussbaum, 2011: x). I argue that this is crucial in thinking about a caring and meaningful education for all children and young people, and indeed it is these points that are the premise of the capabilities approach proposed as a means for thinking through social justice and human rights (Nussbaum, 2011: x). I have identified, in Chapter 2, the ten central Capabilities (Nussbaum, 2011: 33–34) that ought to be enabled in order to ensure a dignified and flourishing life, but the following are particularly pertinent:

- *Affiliation*: live with and towards others and engage in social interaction and have the social bases for self-respect and make provisions for non-discrimination.
- *Play:* being able to laugh, play and enjoy leisure.
- *Control over one's environment*:
  - Political – have the right to participate in political life.
  - Material – have right to seek work, hold property on an equal basis to others.

As Nussbaum's *Affiliation, Play* and *Control over one's environment* suggest, at the very least education ought to be a conduit to affiliating with peers (*Affiliation*), enjoying life (*Play*) and having the opportunity to contribute to or control material and political conditions (*Control over one's environment*). As Nussbaum has suggested, these central capabilities do not presume to solve all distribution problems, but at least propose a significant social minimum for a quality of life, and all ten capabilities are essential conditions of social justice.

I am not going to revisit the problems with a rights-based approach here, as I have discussed this in Chapter 2, but I will recall that despite a rights-based approach being problematic for all concerned in caring, and a care ethics model as such, injustices are not acceptable. Furthermore, I am reminded that we exist in a pluralistic society, and I am not the first, nor will I be the last, to engage with theories that sometimes make us wince in mapping their foundations. As it is, 'exploring the multiplicities of human life can bring great pleasure; but the downside of this is that we have to live with the potential for perpetual conflicts and violence over these differences' (Plummer, 2015: 14), and this includes the theoretical as well as empirical. However, this does not mean we are unable to understand particular social phenomena, and in this case caring in education. As it is, Young (1999: 59, emphasis in original) has suggested that late modern societies '*consume* diversity; they do not recoil at difference, they recast it as a commodity'. Therefore, it is fine to be different, but not difficult. He goes on to say that what many people in modern society are less willing to 'endure is *difficulty*'. This is important here because, for example, Brian, a boy with Down's syndrome in Allan's (1999a) research, was looked upon affectionately because he was different, but not necessarily difficult *per se*. In Benjamin's (2002) research, Josie, who was identified with 'special needs', was difficult as she had additional unruly behaviour, and she was eventually excluded from her mainstream school. These findings are not dissimilar from those of Gillies and Robinson (2010, 2013), who conducted research with 'excluded' young men in schools who were considered difficult and almost uneducable.

Significantly, the late modern world 'celebrates diversity and *difference*, which it readily absorbs and sanitizes; but what it cannot abide is difficult people and *dangerous* classes, which it seeks to build the most elaborate defences against' (Young, 1999: 59). This is critical when thinking about a caring education and inclusion because, although Young (1999) was talking about deviancy and criminality in the research above, it is exclusion and care-less tactics that are a remedy when dealing with difficult differences, whether they are disabled others who are difficult to teach, difficult uncontrollable others, or culturally diverse others who are difficult to understand (within a particular set of cultural norms). In Young's later work he asks us to think about 'othering' and 'elsewhere' in response to differences, and whilst his thesis on late modernity moves towards a blurring of boundaries rather than a binary position of inclusion/exclusion, we are still left with a 'fake sense of solidarity' in celebrating the 'inferior' (Young, 2007: 197) (see also Davis' 2013, work on diversity for a nuanced position on the end of normal). It could be argued that some of this retreat from difficulty, and denial of disability or othering is based on ignorance, on fear (Furedi, 2006), on potential association or on shame (Goffman, 1990). Nussbaum discusses shame and claims that it is ubiquitous and that most of us learn to cover our weakness (2004: 173), and therefore remove ourselves from a shameful experience. This shaming happens all the time for intellectually disabled children within their inhumane and care-less education process.

Nussbaum goes on to maintain that 'modern liberal societies can make adequate response to the phenomena of shame only if they shift away from a very common intuitive idea of the normal citizen that has been bequeathed to us by the social-contract tradition' (2004: 177). Shame is clearly a sense of failure to attain, and is largely based on feelings of inadequacy, including feelings of (or association with) a lack of perfection (Goffman, 1990; Miller, 1997). None of this is attractive, and in the twenty-first century many will withdraw from the very association with 'failure', shame or stigma. As I have already argued, this is not helped by the privileging of educational attainment that, for example, largely depends on scores as a result of examinations that do little more than test memory (Slee, 2011). Education, however, ought to focus on the 'needs and anxieties of the inner self, at the same time developing the capacity to perceive need in others' (Nussbaum, 2004: 203) rather than rote learning (Smyth, Down and McInerney, 2010; see also Allan, 2005), so, a caring and relational education. Nussbaum suggests the government, and I would argue the socio-political sphere that is wider than government, ought not to humiliate but instead work with giving people dignity. For example, it seems that for intellectually disabled people it could be argued that national and global inclusive policies satisfy the need to educate everyone. Yet, in the main, 'we do not treat a child with Down Syndrome in a manner commensurate with that child's dignity if we fail to develop the child's powers of mind through suitable education'. In fact for intellectually disabled people we need to think about policies that support, care and protect rather than infantilise and 'treat them as passive recipients of benefit' (Nussbaum, 2011: 30).

Education is seen as pivotal to the development and exercise of many other human capabilities (Nussbaum, 2011: 152), especially as illiteracy *anywhere* is an enduring disability – which in itself is an injustice and inhumane. As

I argued in the previous chapter, intellectual disability is not *just* about inclusion, but about a whole host of re-humanising processes. We do indeed need a scheme of social cooperation (Nussbaum, 2011: 150), and the inclusion of children in classrooms with other children is crucial (Nussbaum, 2006: 413) to working towards social inclusion. Being critical of the status quo in the current climate is difficult, but Smyth, Down and McInerney (2010), with regards to education, suggest that being committed to change with an emphasis on relationships, pedagogy, school organisation and school-community engagement is crucial if we are to hope for utopia and social transformation, and to eradicate exclusion.

A way forward: re-humanising education

Social justice, relationality, care and ethics need to be considered when exploring intellectual disability, education, inclusion and being human. These aspects, it could be argued, are the basis for a socially inclusive society and a care ethics model of disability. An education that starts with enabling human flourishing and care is essential, because '[b]eing deprived of the capacity to develop supportive affective relations of love, care and solidarity [...] is [...] a serious human deprivation for most people: it is a core dimension of affective inequality' (Lynch, Baker and Lyons, 2009: 1). Moreover, as research suggests, care, especially in early childhood education, is a crucial part of the learning process (Luff, 2013). So thinking about caring and ethics rather than necessarily the pedagogical process is illuminating and essential. In addition, learning ought to take place within and through relationships, and these relationships are critical in developing a healthy sense of self-identity.

Broadly speaking, then, we ought to be who we want to be, as defined by Nussbaum (2011) in pursuing a capabilities approach. We should be able to live in a care-full, moral and ethical environment, as developed and mapped within a care ethics model of disability, without feeling alienated or disengaged (Marx, 2007; Oliver, 1990). Moreover, we ought not to be overly governed and surveyed (Allan, 1999a, 2010a; Foucault, 1991; Slee, 2011), which is particularly pertinent for education and learning. Thus, rather than following a path of blame, whether it is the dysfunctional family, the deficit child or the economically deprived nation, we require ethically just practices and caring as a fundamental part of re-humanised education. Authors such as Smyth, Down and McInerney (2010: 26) argue that 'the poor' are not the problem, thereby dismissing the view that poor families necessarily need to change or that teachers need to 'save' the disadvantaged students. They suggest that the neoliberal lens, where 'we can all succeed in life if we apply ourselves', is far too simplistic and 'downright false'. Significantly, if young people are not able to form relationships they then disconnect, disengage and subsequently 'drop out' of education, and we all suffer as a consequence. The position taken in Smyth, Down and McInerney's (2010) research is that if you trust and respect the young learner to make decisions, then they will generally respond positively.

Of course it is never that simple (Gillies and Robinson, 2010, 2013), but ethical caring, trust and respect are, nevertheless, tantamount in developing a healthy learning environment.

Schools absolutely need risk taking, innovation and experimentation, without which creativity is unable to flourish. Yet we exist within a risk society where no or low risk is positioned as the only way, and we are indeed frightened of risky business, the unknown or litigation (Bauman, 2007; Beck, 1992; Furedi, 2006). So from Gypsy and Traveller children and their exclusion to parents of intellectually disabled children, from pupils gaining participatory voice to support structures being in place, an ethics of care is required (Rose, 2010). To overcome some of these difficulties, Rose suggests a holistic and co-ordinated approach that addresses the cultural, political and socio-economic barriers that maintain the circumstances within which many of the world's population live in poverty and experience marginalisation while the gap widens between those with and those without. Crucially for this work, some of the obstacles to inclusion and a care-full education are so deeply embedded and prolific within the socio-political sphere, for example as in the case of media representations of disability, that much more care-full work needs to continue. Furthermore, the difficulty in many of the current narratives, whether on the screen or in policy discourses, are often couched within a medical model and at best place disabled people within a heroic discourse, but ultimately they are positioned as 'less than human' (Rose, 2010: 16), as has been the case for decades:

> Many of our schools are in what might be called a crisis of caring. Both students and teachers are brutally attacked verbally and physically. Clearly, the schools are not often places where caring is fulfilled, but it is not always the failure of teachers that causes the lapse in caring. […] No matter what they do, it seems, their efforts are not perceived as caring. They themselves are perceived, instead, as the enemy, as natural targets for resistance.
>
> (Noddings, 2003[1984]: 181)

This quote, albeit over three decades old now, is relevant today, as is clear from the research discussed above and the narratives I have identified. It is time to apply a care ethics model of disability to education that includes all caring spheres, and all humans, but this cannot be done in a vacuum. Therefore it makes sense to look to the family, and mainly mothering, as I have identified already that domestic relations are key in working towards both a caring and care-full education and a caring and care-full domestic environment. While the following chapter is very different in many ways, by looking at care-less spaces via mothering, the development of a caring narrative is, I hope, evident. Ultimately we all need to be mindful that when addressing a caring and ethical education there will always be a care-full or care-less (or something in between) environment beyond the school gate, and more often than not the home. This is why no one area can work alone in mapping a care ethics model of disability.

Notes

1 Of course I recognise '[t]he hooligan, defective, feeble-minded and delinquent loafers of 1910 have become the yobs, chavs, NEETS and scroungers of 2010' (Tomlinson, 2013: 1), implying that there have always been those who are excluded from meaningful education. But this does not make it right, and there are specific difficulties around those who are unable to engage with a curriculum solely based on reading, writing and examinations.
2 The DfES existed until 2007, and was then replaced, in part by the Department for Children, Schools and Families (DCSF), until the coalition government came into power in 2010. It then became the Department for Education (DfE).
3 A–C grade at GCSE (General Certificate in Secondary Education) are considered the appropriate academic national standards in England, Wales and Northern Ireland for going on to study after the age of 16. They also identify schools that maintain a particular academic standard and those that do not within the league table system. But this of course does not tell the story of intellectual disability, except that these students are missing, literally and metaphorically.
4 Children in England, Wales and Northern Ireland usually aged 14–16 in years 10 and 11.
5 SATs is a common term for statutory assessment tests or national curriculum educational assessments which are tests carried out in schools at the age of 7 and 11. Until 2009 children were also tested via this route at the age of 14.
6 This is explored in Chapter 4.
7 Between 2014 and 2018, changes are implemented to the statementing process. Education Health and Care Plans (EHCs) are a new form of assessment. That said, thus far, mechanisms of support and care-full practices have not been rolled out sufficiently.
8 Rhizome is a concept developed by Deleuze and Guattari (see Allan, 2010a). It is about non-hierarchical knowledge. It could be likened metaphorically to a rabbit warren or an ant colony, where new ways of going (or thinking, in the case of philosophy, sociology and politics) are potentially there to pursue.
9 This might seem trite to those living and dealing with disability and impairments every day, but it is meant to respond to the wider cultural context of consumerism, individualism, therapeutic discourse and a pursuit of perfection – which is unattainable.

4 Mothering and (in)humanity: care-less spaces

Listening to BBC Radio 4 the Today show this morning on 15 July 2014, Sara Ryan's voice crosses the airwaves just over a year after Connor's death (Connor was her son). He was an 18-year-old autistic young man, with a rare syndrome and epilepsy. Understandably her voice cracks as she talks about her son's tragic and preventable death in an NHS assessment and treatment unit. She tells the listener that the fight for justice has been a distraction and the support, as well as the knowledge that many people feel so enraged, gives her comfort. Of course every day that passes will not bring her son back. The unit that Connor was in has now since been closed, but we are still talking about death and abuse over three years since the Winterbourne case and the British government promised a reduction in these assessment unit placements. The number has risen. Death feels (is) final. As I listened to the programme one father discusses how he travels for 7 hours to see his 12-year-old autistic son who is in one of these 'care' units. His son has been there for two years. It might be too late for Connor, but justice and caring practices can be served, as we urge for ethical care within a care ethics model of disability and stop other abuse and preventable deaths for intellectually disabled people. I think about Connor, my own adult intellectually disabled daughter and all the other Dudes (as Sara would say).

(personal reflections, July 2014)

Introduction: the mother speaks first

This introductory quote, from my personal reflections, and the lengthy narratives below, present different versions of, and responses to, mothering and intellectual disability. They capture an everyday life, but they also afford us a glimpse into the broader and more violent emotional, practical and socio-political caring spheres, or care-less spaces around us. That is to say, not only do mothers and fathers with an intellectually disabled child have a deeply emotional response to their lived experiences, but the legal, moral and political systems also disturb, and can ultimately destroy lives without caring, which can include education processes but is not limited to these exclusively as they leak into the family, domestic sphere and more 'private' domains. Just as in the previous chapter I found rhetoric within education discourse, the mother and others caring are amongst those who are also 'cared for', apparently. As it is, the

> well-dressed businessman with his rights of autonomy; freedom, of contract; and presumption of innocence can be well advised by our law graduates. The exhausted mother of the disabled child, with little autonomy, freedom or innocence, cannot. She is an anomaly, outside the norm. Not even, perhaps, of particular interest to lawyers. After all she will not be able to pay any fees. *Yet everyone cares. Everyone is cared for.*
>
> (Herring, 2013: 1; emphasis added)

Thus, I reflect on Sara Ryan's story here (as well as others) as her personal circumstances have touched many lives, and as someone who knows her as a fellow academic and a mother, it seems fitting to remember Connor, or Laughing Boy (LB), as he was known.

The all-encompassing socio-political sphere, and within that the legal system, has been care-less. The quote below, from Sara Ryan's public blog, is about the immediate aftermath of the death of her son, who was 'in care' for a little over three months after being sectioned. I might have assumed he was in a caring and care-full space. It seemed he was not, as evidenced here.

> As I've probably banged on about before, I can't stand this 'give people voice' crap. It's so patronising and offensive it makes my ears weep. People have voices (or other ways of communicating). They don't need to be given them. The problems here don't lie with learning disabled people not having 'voices'. They lie with people not listening. Not understanding. And not *caring*. [...] I don't think people will really start to care properly until they see learning disabled people as full and valued members of society. At a micro level, LB (laughing boy) was valued. There has been an enormous response to his death which has been a source of some comfort. People seem genuinely upset and angered by what happened to him. A happening in which he had no 'choice' or 'voice', or other crap like that. This upset and anger has come about because people got to know him as a person, as a funny young man who had a refreshing approach to life. [...] People said for years said I should write about LB; he was such a hilarious dude. I started this blog partly as a way of recording these funny stories. I didn't anticipate it would be widely read. Or that it would take such a terrible, terrible direction. [...] Not every dude like LB will have someone to write their story (if they can't do it themselves). We need to find other ways of making people care. Of accepting and celebrating learning disabled people as fully human And then maybe the government wouldn't baulk at the 'cost' of setting up a review board to investigate how and why these deaths are occurring. But then, of course, they probably wouldn't happen with such regularity.
>
> (Ryan, 2013c)

I can, in an instant, feel the enormity of care-lessness, care lack, and how voices that are *real representations* of people are missing, or indeed talked about in an utterly meaningless way. These are not the representations we see in the popular media that are discussed throughout the book. This young man had no part to play in his death, and existed within a care-less space, where emotional, practical and socio-political damage was executed. Tragic as this is, what Sara is asking, or rather stating, in her blog is, 'who will speak up for intellectually disabled people if M(O)thers do not?' In considering this, I need to situate the mother, the one caring, in an interdependent relationship, but one that also involves the emotional, practical and socio-political caring spheres.

In another example of how mothers experience their position as a care-full or caring mother, I reflect on the work of John Vorhaus (2016). He identifies Emily Kingsley's 'Welcome to Holland', as Emily likens having a disabled child to landing in the wrong destination after booking, planning and packing for a trip to Italy. Emily metaphorically lands in Holland. Not what she expected, but says 'if you spend your life mourning the fact that you didn't get to Italy, you may never be free to enjoy the very special, the very lovely things ... about Holland' (Vorhaus, 2016: 116). Vorhaus (2016) discusses this in some detail, but goes on to suggest that not all parents share Emily's sentiment. As it is, Vorhaus starkly compares this with Cheryl Arvidson-Keating's piece called 'Welcome to Fucking Holland'. This is in response to her daughter who has significant and multiple impairments; the contrast in attitude is striking. Cheryl is discussing in her written piece how little respite is available, and after a few days away without her daughter, she reflects

> I am so bloody tired of everything. Five child-free days in Toulouse was wonderful ... Coming home and here I am again... all I want to do is escape, either physically, or in to my head... [...] everything revolves around her [...] I resent that I have a future that involves changing adult nappies and using a bath-lift and knackering my back lifting someone who doesn't have muscle control. [...] I resent the fact that my beautiful, clever, funny, amazing daughter, who I love so much it hurts, is not going to have the life that she should have had; and that we will not have the life we should have had with her. I resent the fact that our entire fucking life has been hijacked by one measly gene fragment that doesn't even have the decency to be easily found. Welcome to fucking Holland. It's shit here.
>
> (Vorhaus, 2016: 117)

Vorhaus is making a point in contrasts, but also recognising that this life, the disabled life, the caring and care-full life, is hard and indeed often care-less. For the one caring as well as the intellectually disabled person. He also goes on to identify that Cheryl writes a retrospective piece about how she felt she had to go through that dark depressive place as she hit 'rock bottom' as a way of coming to terms with everything that goes on in mothering a profoundly disabled 'child'. The point is, that if Cheryl had been in a different caring space when at her darkest moment, a different outcome might have occurred. Of course, this is unknowable, yet what we can know is that care-full spaces are always necessary, or tragic circumstances can occur.

The following narratives are from my research data. Importantly, as with Vorhaus's (2016) work, they situate how we understand mothering in the context of emotional responses to rearing a child who is intellectually disabled and how everyday prejudice occurs via others' care-less reactions to intellectually disabled children within an institutional and emotional context. I already identified the care-less space in the playground in Chapter 2 (see in detail Rogers, 2013c) and Francis, a mother with a son who has Asperger syndrome, told me in a previous interview, 'a few years ago I thought, that's it. You can keep him, I don't want him, I just want some peace in my life'. Furthermore, Tracy, talking about one of her disabled sons who has cerebral palsy, said of his first day at school:

> So the first day at school came and they had their little uniforms on and I walked them up to the school [...] I came back to pick them up at the end of the day and erm, as I walked into the playground the teacher went (she beckoned) like to me and the headmistress went (the same) and I went over to her and she said 'into my office please'. I thought they can't have been naughty like that on the first day! She got me in her office; she said 'take a seat' – she's curt – (and Tracy mimicked this) 'I wasn't aware I was having a bloody retard in my school' [...] I went mental, absolutely mental... [...] So I went mental and ended up with the police coming round [...] Me getting arrested [...] I got to the stage where I thought I was a completely lousy mother and they'd be better off without me anyway [...] I was getting to the stage where they would be better off without me. But I suppose it was them that kept me on an even keel so to speak.

In addition, recall from Chapter 1 my own attempts at blogging, when my intellectually disabled daughter was misidentified as a perpetrator of a criminal act, subsequently arrested, charged, held in a police cell and interviewed. This had incredibly negative impacts and was systemically violent.

In all the narratives acknowledged in this opening, where the mother speaks first, there is an array of imagery on how we might attempt to understand the emotional, practical and socio-political caring spheres that are, namely, care-less spaces; carelessness in the school, playground, health care system, criminal justice system, and so on. Again, as with the quote from Tracy, we can see the institutional carelessness being played out. Moreover it is a care-less space across all of the caring spheres, the emotional, the practical and the socio-political, as all relate to each other in complex ways. Ultimately, there is a procedural carelessness, like with the internal and external reviews that have taken place for Connor Sparrowhawk (Justice for LB, 2015a). Also at a basic level, I was told, as a result of the internal review of my daughter's arrest, 'we did everything by the book, and in fact your daughter was treated very well, after all we wouldn't usually let another adult in the cell with a detainee'. They did indeed allow my husband, her stepfather, into the cell, but this inspector was at that time talking about a 27-year-old intellectually disabled woman, who was clearly distressed, innocent and cognitively unable to process why she was there, and I, as her mother, was supposed to be grateful they apparently 'bent the rules'. We know, too well, that many more tragic stories have been told by those who were following orders (Bauman, 1989).

The final quote in this extended introduction, 'the mother speaks first', is from philosopher Eva Kittay about the ugliness and animality of intellectual disability. As a philosopher and a mother with an adult intellectually disabled daughter, Kittay says,

> [i]magine being the mother of a child with severe intellectual disabilities reading within the pages of a philosophical text such statements as: "I have argued that the cognitively impaired are not badly off in the sense relevant to justice [...] Not only do they not have special priority as a matter of justice, but their claims on us seem even weaker than those of most other human beings" [....] "the treatment of animals is governed by stronger constraints than we have traditionally supposed, while the treatment of the cognitively impaired is in some respects subject to weaker constraints" [...] For a mother of a severely cognitively impaired child, the impact of such an argument is devastating. How can I begin to tell you what it feels like to read texts in which one's child is compared, in all seriousness and with philosophical authority, to a dog, pig, rat, and most flatteringly a chimp; how corrosive these comparisons are, how they mock those relationships that affirm who we are and why we care?
>
> (Kittay, 2010: 396–397)

Without a doubt these opening narratives from mothers identify that mothering under extreme circumstances is difficult, if not at times unbearable, and that it can cause suffering. As Martha Nussbaum (who has a disabled nephew) says, '[p]arents are reproved for allowing such a child to come into existence; the whole life of such children has been regarded as an ugly mistake' (Nussbaum, 2004: 306). The suffering, disquiet, reflection and anger talked about in all of these narratives manifests in emotional and physical cruelty, systemic violence and abject governance, and is based on care-less and inhumane legal and moral positions, best interests and a 'worthy' life. It is for these reasons that I want to talk about the dark side of mothering and to propose a care ethics model of disability as a way forward, as *no one* ought to suffer as a human being through mothering their intellectually disabled child.

Mothering and a care-less context

Another year on from the personal reflection above (5 July 2015), and two years and a day after Connor Sparrowhawk's death, I viewed a video online about the death of Connor, or Laughing Boy (LB) as he is more commonly known. It was moving, celebratory and yet stark; stark in the telling of a care-less story about the meaningless death of a young man inhabiting a care-less space. Connor's mother, Sara Ryan, his stepfather, siblings, friends and others caring, all reminisce. This painful but care-full narrative speaks volumes, and as Sara speaks for her laughing boy she does so for all intellectually disabled people. She movingly says in the video,

> My beyond wildest dreams would be that – we are never going to achieve this in a million years – but would be that we didn't even have to talk about learning disabled people, because, because there wouldn't need to be that division, because everybody would have a right to live where they choose, everybody has an imagined future, and the distinction between being learning disabled and being non-learning disabled would become sort of irrelevant because it isn't an issue. That, that I suppose is my wildest dream, but whether that will happen or not, I, I don't know, so we'll reach for the stars and see what happens. Coz I think Connor's up there.
>
> (Ryan, 2015)

This might seem too much to ask, but if we collectively do not reach for the stars, aim for a caring, care-full and humane society, then we do not have hope.

Genuinely, this mothering chapter has been the hardest one to write because, as you know by now, I am a mother with an adult intellectually disabled daughter. I also know mothers who have intellectually disabled children as friends, family and acquaintances, and the personal is political and philosophical. Also, as the reader will be aware, from the opening and just above, tragically, Sara Ryan, who is a close fellow academic, is writing a public blog and campaigning about the avoidable death of her son, as well as those of others. Appallingly this is yet another 'death by indifference' (Bawden and Campbell, 2012; Goldring, 2012; Mencap, 2007, 2012), in the UK alone, and not the most recent either. Intellectually disabled people continue to die because of delays in diagnosis, failure to recognise pain, messiness around 'do not resuscitate' (DNR), mental capacity issues, lack of basic care and poor communication (Mencap, 2012). This violence continues despite the fact that a document in 2007 highlighted avoidable deaths of intellectually disabled people (Mencap, 2007). Avoidable deaths and systemic violence also manifest, albeit to the extreme, when a mother kills her intellectually disabled child and then commits suicide.

Cases about killing children include that of Joanne Hill, who was jailed for drowning her four-year-old daughter who had cerebral palsy (Hornby, 2008);

Ajit Singh-Mahal, who admitted killing her 12-year-old autistic son and then attempting to take her own life (BBC News, 2010); and Fiona Pilkington, who took her own life and that of her 18-year-old disabled daughter, due, according to her diaries, to persistent harassment from local young people (Walker, 2009). Stories like these have also been highlighted in television broadcasts, with Rosa Monckton's 'Tormented Lives' shown in 2010 on the BBC, depicting mothers who experience everyday abuse and exclusion, alongside the more mundane day-to-day care practices with their disabled children. Mothers interviewed by Monckton told her how there were times when life was ulti-mately not worth living, that life was so full of carelessness that the choices between life and death became blurred. This too has been highlighted in my research narratives, as one mother told me about how she just wanted to 'take a bottle of pills' (see Rogers 2007a, 2013a). None of these women, in Monckton's broadcast or interviewed as part of my research, necessarily experienced depression or mental health difficulties prior to this particular experience of mothering a disabled child. The sheer social and emotional drain, and the suffering, compounded by the lack of caring networks, care-less spaces and negative social attitudes, seemed too much to bear at times (see also Vorhaus, 2016).

As preposterous as a mother taking the life of her child might seem, one could argue it is an example of extreme caring, where they are relieving themselves and their child of the everyday disabling conditions and experi-ences of care-lessness. How can we live in such an inhumane, care-less and unjust society, where taking a life, your child's life, is a way out? Moreover, utter despair is experienced by mothers because no service, network or support is envisaged as a way to end suffering. I can see this in all of the narratives above, whether in a mother feeling emotionally drained, in need of some peace, and at odds with institutional structures and care-less humans, or in relation to the broader, more philosophical lack of care that impacts upon the socio-political sphere and the psycho-social. The enormity of caring, care-full work and emotional work that some mothers carry out as a part of their mothering is at times considered unbearable. What the examples above demonstrate are that in extreme cases, the caring and emotional work involved can go against culturally accepted norms of a mother taking care of her child unconditionally and keeping them alive. Yet, I would argue that this extreme form of caring – death, in fact murder – is indeed carried out in the name of extreme love or caring, or as a result of desperation and suffering. Such extreme cases might cause us to question what is 'natural', for example, about killing a child, including whether this can be considered caring, moral or ethical. Indeed, is it caring and ethical to suggest that the caring work carried out with and for a disabled (and/or 'difficult') child is done so out of necessity or obligation rather than love (Nutt, 2013)? Tracy, one of my research parti-cipants, told me 'only a mother could actually put up with this' (care-lessness and enormous caring work) and 'there are certain things in life where you haven't got a choice'. Caring and ethics, in this sense, could be about human frailty and vulnerability, as is implied by Tracy when she asks who else will do it, who else will be caring and care-full.

Intellectually disabled children are at times both vulnerable and frail, and therefore unable to care for themselves. Nevertheless, the mother is also frail and vulnerable at times during her maternal journey. This is why a care ethics model of disability is necessary, as all of these caring relations are inter-dependent. Moreover, they include the three spheres of caring I have outlined throughout. Interestingly, Noddings (1995: 9) talks about the relationship between 'natural' and 'ethical' caring as it is often considered that mothering and a 'mother's love' are 'natural' and caring, but that caring is also moral and ethical, and often fraught with conflict, as already identified (see Tronto, 1993a, 1993b). This particular killing field is philosophically a very dangerous place to go. All human lives are worth living, and all are worthy of humanity and caring. Thus, when stories of a mother killing her disabled child are portrayed in the media or an intellectually disabled young adult dies prematurely 'in care', moral and ethical questions need to asked and answered. These might be about the care of the child, the mother's mental health, or the carelessness experienced by such families from external agencies and wider society.

In a less extreme example, Mumsnet (2013), a blogging site tagged 'By Parents, For Parents', has opened a space for mothers with intellectually disabled children, or those identified with 'special education needs' (SEN). This is largely due to problems around dealing with discovering a child's impairment, 'special education', education professionals, inclusion and assessments. Mumsnet is a hugely classed space but some mothers are blogging about their everyday lives, which has become a pastime and a place for gaining answers to questions about their children generally, but it has also been suggested that it is a space to care and do care-full work (Doucet and Mauthner, 2013). Doucet and Mauthner are engaging in critical debate, and do ask questions of 'mommy blogging' in relation to this 'caring space' as they ponder the separation of care, work and consumption practices, as well as questioning how integrated or distinct from care work it is (Doucet and Mauthner, 2013: 103). Nevertheless, people in different blogging and Internet forums come together to discuss issues virtually and often with a view to supporting and caring for one another. For example, Sara Ryan, in her *mydaftlife* blogs, has had hugely compassionate and care-full responses since her 'death post'. Therefore, in life and in death there are necessary discussions to be had about intellectual disability, mothering, care and being human, as I discuss below.

Caring in life and death: can we hope?

Thinking further about caring and suffering, Hooyman and Gonyea (1999) make a useful distinction between caring *for* and caring *about*, suggesting that 'caring about implies affection and perhaps a sense of psychological responsibility, whereas caring for encompasses both the performance or supervision of concrete tasks and a sense of psychological responsibility' (Hooyman and

Gonyea 1999: 151). This is an important distinction to make in thinking about how to alleviate suffering via humane action, as well as in thinking about how we manage care emotionally, practically and politically. Research carried out by Kathleen Lynch (2007) and her colleagues (Lynch, Baker and Lyons, 2009) provides a comprehensive understanding of care and love. Lynch (2007) suggests that there are three spheres of care: love labouring, general care work and solidarity work. Significantly here for the mother and her emotive response is Lynch's (2007) notion of love labouring, or the care given by the primary carer which is intimate in nature, and in this case may refer to the mother's emotional work. But 'general care work' is also important as it is associated with secondary care relations; so extended family relations, neighbours and friendship networks. Moreover, however, 'solidarity work', which forms part of tertiary care relations or public care work, is critical as it is here that the broader socio-cultural and socio-political spheres are influential (Lynch, 2007: 562). I find this really useful in proposing a care ethics model of disability, but in this instance via three spheres of caring – emotional, practical and socio-political.

Critically, practical caring *and* love labouring can cause immense distress, and in some cases induce suffering for mothers, arising from the extreme emotional labour carried out but also due to systemic violence and carelessness politically. Consider the excerpt from Sara's blog early in the chapter. Sara, a sociologist and mother with an intellectually disabled son, Connor, started her blog when he was 17 years old. My understanding of it was that it was largely about the desire to be lighthearted in narrating living with disability, principally because the records of so many lives recounted (my research included) paint depressing and often harrowing tales. Sara, on the other hand, wanted to share the 'fun stuff', as well as have a 'record of random happenings that I've experienced over time' as she put it. Nevertheless, all good intentions aside, it also became about 'the experience of negotiating mental health/learning disability services, as the lack of both meant that LB (Connor) was admitted to inpatient care a few months ago now' (Ryan, 2013a). In March 2013, at the beginning of the care-less 'in care' story, Sara tells us her son has been sectioned and 'it's easy to pop in for 10 minutes and the open door policy gives some confidence in how the staff are treating the patients'. Yet negotiating the services was tragically only the tip of the iceberg regarding this story, as, in July 2013, Connor was found dead in the bath. The tale that Sara, or any other mother, does not want to tell, ever, is that of the meaningless and preventable death of her child. Sara's death and grieving story, like others (Mencap, 2012), is about care-less, moral and ethical lack: lack of communication, caring and humanity, prior to, during and after a tragic event. Particularly here, care-lessness is evident within the socio-political sphere, where institutional processes attempt to manage a difficulty like the inconvenience of a puncture in a tyre. Damage limitation and patching it up seemed to be the initial response, and indeed ongoing narrative. But this carelessness is much less obvious in the immediate emotional sphere and psycho-socially, where narrating the death and subsequent events aids public resolve and, with the help of social media, thousands rally and support this particular mothering. Importantly here, for stories such as Sara's and those of other mothers who have lost their children through such things as negligence, lack of caring, incompetence and so on (Mencap, 2007, 2012), Jane Ribbens McCarthy (2013) talks about caring after death in a different, but nevertheless useful context, from that of disability.

In Ribbens McCarthy's research, she discusses the person left behind, the body of the living, where 'grief and loss may be experienced as a physical pain in one's own body' (2013: 184), and where embodied relationality highlights one of the deep paradoxes in the costs and benefits of caring that arise when we recognise how individual well-being and flourishing may be bound up with that of others (Ribbens McCarthy, 2013: 184). So, bound in every way imaginable with a person, for example, a mother and her intellectually disabled 'child', the death is physically and emotionally beyond words. As Sara posted on the day of LB's death, 'LB died this morning. In the bath. In the unit. He would be pleased the CID are involved'. And the day after, on the 5 July 2013, she posted:

> I made sounds at the hospital yesterday I never expected to make. Or even knew I could make. Sounds of keening, howling, inconsolable, incomprehensible grief, sorrow, despair and darkness. Our beautiful, hilarious, exceptional dude was found unconscious in the bath in the unit before a planned trip [...]. The psychiatrist from the unit who called me at work around 10am to say that LB had been taken to hospital, gave no steer he was pretty much dead. I asked her (as an anxiety induced afterthought) if he was conscious when he left the unit in the ambulance. She said they'd cleared his airway but he hadn't regained consciousness. She made no suggestion I should urgently go to the hospital or that I should go with someone. It was a *care less* call. [...]. I arrived at the hospital twenty or so minutes later, with a work colleague who (so, so kindly) insisted on coming with me. I was immediately faced with a LB has a 'dead heart only kept alive by a ventilator' story. This news generated my, to that point, unknown sounds. I hugged him while he died. Unspeakable horror. Agonising pain. [...] We are now in a space I can't describe. [...] I can't move beyond wondering how a hospital unit, with only four or five patients, who made such a fucking fuss about asking LB's permission for us to visit on a daily basis, could let him die in the bath.
>
> (Ryan, 2013b, emphasis added)

This physical and emotional reaction to the death of someone so close is common, as Ribbens McCarthy (2013: 190) states in relation to being told of her husband's imminent death: 'At this point I felt as if someone had lobbed an axe into my chest and that I was then expected to carry on walking around in the world with an axe in my chest and tears pouring down my face'. This talk of death, followed by the actual suffering experienced, might seem extreme; after all, many parents do not experience their 'child's' death, but the point here, in talking about this, is that it absolutely highlights how we understand suffering. It seems therefore appropriate, within a care ethics model of disability, to turn to Frank (2001: 355), who explains that loss and suffering (whether present or anticipated) is an 'instance of no thing, an absence of what was missed and now is no longer recoverable and the absence of what we fear will never be'. Bureaucratic processes cannot manage this suffering; bureaucratic processes are care-less. Yet we need them to be care-full, ethical and humane, and if we bring together the emotional, practical and sociopolitical caring spheres in an ethical manner we can attempt to make change. Yet even in care-full spaces there will be human suffering. Like with education in the previous chapter, in discussing the need for creativity, it might be that we also need creative care-full spaces in suffering.

As it is, in loss narratives the physical meets the emotional, as I reflect, for example, in my own miscarriage story (Rogers, 2009b: 97). As I lost the second foetus I said to my husband:

> 'Look at this'; I held it out in the palm of my hands [...]. I sobbed and sobbed. My heart was so broken I didn't think I would survive: the emotional pain so sharp, so deep [...] It was bleak and a long moment that took me outside of any rational thoughts *per se*. I needed freedom from that. It was black Thursday for me. The 28th January was the darkest day I could ever remember. I lay in bed.... Nothing but despair. Actually nothing at all. But this was interspersed with sobbing. Not a little weep, but proper sobbing. I did wonder if I would ever stop. The day seemed long and so did the next. Time just seemed to have stopped. I know other people's lives would seem like another week had passed by, but for me these few days were eternal. For the first time ever I wondered what it would be like to die: to end this life. I guess not in any real sense, I am still here, but in the sense of ending the emotional pain. I wanted *that* to end.

While the death of a partner or foetus is perhaps incomparable to that of a teenage son or daughter, all of these painful narratives are vivid, haunting and evocative. Therefore, I reduce this to an eschatological event (perhaps extreme, but we are talking about life and death after all) and draw upon Paul Ricoeur's (1995) work.

Ricoeur (1995: 206) proposes that in many ways the personal, collective, ethical and political 'are irreducible to a mere wisdom of the eternal present: they bear the mark of the future – of the "not yet" and of the "much more"; in terms of Kierkegaard, hope makes of freedom the passion for the possible against the sad meditation on the irrevocable'. It is difficult to see how hope can be any part of these loss stories, yet we need hope (as we need caring) as a survival mechanism, and I assert that it is a human trait, an irrefutable part of being human. Indeed, it is arguably necessary in life after suffering. Hope does not have to manifest in the same way for all, and for some it will take different forms throughout various times in life (see Smith and Sparkes, 2005). For Sara and LB, and in the move from the horror of losing a child to a more manageable way of being, this hope, I would argue, has manifested itself via activism and social support, via Twitter (*@justiceforlb*) and local and national interest, and indeed via caring, for example. No raw emotional pain can be eradicated, but collective caring ethics and care-full and humane practice can aid a healthier emotional (psycho-social) state, while impacting upon the socio-political sphere.

Personally, when I think about hope as a mother with an intellectually disabled daughter, I have indeed spent most of her life hoping that she will be okay, just as Sara would have before her son died, just as the mothers in my research, the mothers in my M-CM network, and most other mothers would, with respect to their children, whatever the circumstances (Condry, 2007). I, for example, have often thought over time about my own daughter, 'Will she reach that next milestone?' 'Will she find a loving partner for life?' 'Will she live a long life?' 'Will she have the baby she wants?' 'Will she ever leave home?' More recently, with her MRI scans, diagnosis of Chiari malformation, her everyday symptoms and neurosurgery appointments, I sometimes wake up in the morning asking myself 'Will she be alive?' I can answer these questions with an emphatic 'I hope so', always. Hope at times might seem futile and naïve, but I know that my daughter's hope, that one day she will get married, to the point of planning for it pretty much every day in one way or another, is clearly a crucial coping mechanism in her, some might say, restricted and sometimes care-less life. She may never experience married life. However, we know that many young people expect that they will experience partnership and children (Henderson et al., 2007), so why not my daughter?

Yet hope can be considered unfathomable, unknowable, faith based. Hoping for something suggests that one does not know that it will occur, but that it *might* do. We hope for justice, for care, for humanity, for a meaningful everyday life, yet there is no rational system that we can tap into when it comes to life and loss, where we can say absolutely this will or will not occur. Notably, bringing together philosophical reflection in this way with people's everyday actual experiences, I again look to Ricoeur's work (1989, 1995) and find the notion of hope and a passion for the possible (see Vanhoozer, 1990) in engaging with existence and thinking. That is, existence precedes thinking, not the other way round as in Cartesian philosophy (Vanhoozer, 1990). Actually, for human beings the passion to exist as a basic desire is far more significant in Ricoeur's work (not the nothingness commonly associated with Sartre) (Vanhoozer, 1990). Hope is irrational, but so are life and death. Just as life is not about normalising, standardising and sameness, it is also not rational. Maybe freedom of the passion for the possible can exist and therefore we can all 'hope in order to understand' (Ricoeur, 1995: 207). We can certainly remain hopeful when it comes to proposing a care ethics model of disability, and to exacting change in caring, ethics, social justice and what it means to be a human being. However, hope will not do. Hoping is not doing. Therefore, we need to consider this further, as the 'cost' of mothering and suffering is high and demands attention.

The 'cost' of mothering

In mothering an intellectually disabled child or adult, there are significant costs, as we have seen played out in the above. These costs straddle the emotional, practical and socio-political caring spheres. However, none of these 'caring costs' are easily defined due to the messy nature of the emotional work, love labouring and care work involved. Critically, in thinking about mothering, being human and care ethics, it is important to recognise that expectations during pregnancy and beyond can be full of hopes and dreams for a child's future (albeit in different cultural contexts these expectations might differ). Broadly, mothers often see their child moving towards some kind of independence and autonomy, and quite often believe them to be extensions of themselves (Smart and Neale, 1999: 106). I would argue that all mothers have these hopes, but for some, in extreme circumstances, as in the case of a mother who sees her son imprisoned for murder or rape (Condry, 2007), these hopes are ruptured, tainted, if not ruined. No mother rears her child and thinks s/he will kill or rape another human, just as she does assume, or at least hope, her child will read, write and have a full and flourishing life. An intellectually disabled child's impairment will often fracture dreams and is often in conflict with hopeful expectations; for example, an autistic child who is unable to communicate cannot necessarily be an extension of the mother's self without invoking angst about what that self is. Or a child with Down's syndrome may be unable to negotiate full independence, autonomy or separateness, and thereby challenge a mother's notion of successfully mothering a fully independent young adult. Despite considering interdependence, rather than independence, emotionally this does not fully compute when contemplating a child's future and their life long journey. Therefore, it has been found, mothers are often left wondering about their own future and how their caring persona (potentially) spills over into their old age as their child becomes a dependent or interdependent adult (Barnes, 2006; Bowlby et al., 2010).

Indeed, this is just the tip of the iceberg when it comes to moderate and severe intellectual disability. Undeniably these dashed hopes and emotional and practical costs feed the notion that disability is a burden to both the individual and society, straddling the emotional, practical and socio-political spheres. It is because of this very notion that a care ethics model of disability is crucial, and that this disability 'burden' is recognised and discussed via discourses on, for example, human need (Dean, 2010), capabilities (Nussbaum, 2011; Sen, 2009), social justice and care ethics (Held, 1995, 2006; Lynch, Baker and Lyons, 2009), genetics and the 'worthy' life (Kittay, 2005, 2010; Pfeiffer, 2006; Shakespeare, 2006). To be sure, we need to understand the *value* of care and care-full support for families and their intellectually disabled children.

Moreover, we need to provide a platform for understanding interdependence, with a view to promoting socially just practices and alleviating suffering (McLaughlin et al., 2008; Nussbaum, 2006). Critically, a feminist ethics of care problematises care in relation to, for example, the capacity to care, caring relations, gendered practice, labour, autonomy and dependence (see for example, Held, 1995, 2006; Lynch, Baker and Lyons, 2009; Tronto, 1993a, 1993b). Some disability literature, in a different way, has been very critical of interpretations of care and caring practices (see for example, Hughes et al., 2005; Shakespeare, 2006; Thomas, 2007). I understand this aspect from a historical perspective, and practically, but more broadly speaking, disability activists have not always listened to intellectually disabled people, or, more to the point, to those speaking on their behalf. Yes there are different caring issues, but when it comes to thinking about humanity, being human and care ethics, we all want the same thing – to live in humane and care-full conditions, and to be interdependent.

Not all disabled people suffer in the way I am discussing here. Nevertheless, the cost of mothering and intellectual disability can assume some suffering. After all, who would take their child's life if they were not suffering? Yet we know people do. Conversely, the suffering involved in losing a child is unimaginably hard to contemplate. Still, this happens. But according to Wilkinson (2005: 1) suffering is not accepted 'as a normal and inevitable part of our human condition. This is because suffering hurts too much. The problem with suffering is that it involves us in far *too much* pain [...] Suffering destroys our bodies, ruins our minds, and smashes our "spirit"' (emphasis in original). Although within sociological debates suffering is often discussed in terms of *social* suffering, and frequently in relation to mass atrocities (Cohen, 2001; Wilkinson, 2005), it is not exclusively the case, as suffering is a 'deeply personal experience' (Wilkinson, 2005: 16), so it can be difficult to understand socially. It also has the potential to damage every aspect of personhood. Certainly in dying people suffer acute emotional pain and, as Wilkinson (2005: 17) suggests, suffering is 'always against us'. Suffering might always feel care-less, but how we respond to it, socially, ethically and politically, and collectively need not.

Critically, Wilkinson (2005: 3) insists that sociological research often ignores what the actual '*experience* of suffering *does* to people' (emphasis in original) and, what is more, the lived experience is rarely the direct focus. However, he does point out that sociological research is more often than not about suffering, for example, poverty, injustice, exclusion, abuse, to name just a few. Frank (1995, 2001), as discussed above, also discusses suffering. He draws on Cassell's three conditions of suffering; in short, the conditions of suffering involve the whole person, suffering takes place within a state of severe distress, and it occurs in relation to any aspect of the person (Frank, 1995: 170). Frank adds to Cassell's conditions a fourth and fifth, which are *resistance* and its *social nature*. I would argue that his fourth condition is crucial as he proposes *telling stories* as a form of resistance. So, for example, if we suffer, the telling of the story, writing a blog, re-telling the story to a researcher, or diary writing, poetry, or letter writing, can also act as a form of resistance to suffering (or carefulness) and indeed, meaning-making processes that can then invoke hopeful narratives. So what is it in the human condition that makes one come back from such suffering? Of course we could answer this by invoking the simple survival instinct, but as a sociologist and via philosophy, it seems that not all have this ability to move away from things that hurt us, 'voluntarily' or not, as in the case of domestic or sexual violence (Kelly, 1988) and spinal cord injury (Smith and Sparkes, 2005), or in the case of killing your child, as above, for example. Essentially using divine faith, spirituality, or other 'alternative' ways of moving through difficult periods is not unusual, and at times it is narratives of hope which aid in understanding the inexplicable. Therefore it is hardly surprising that sociologists who discuss aging, death and bereavement often hear stories that involve an attempt to understand some kind of afterlife (Earle, Bartholomew and Komaromy, 2009; Ribbens McCarthy, 2013; Woodthorpe, 2011).

Hope, hope-full and care-full narratives also signify a good future, something to aspire to and something to live for, and within different societies this manifests in various ways. Many different cultures and communities use 'hopeful' ceremonies as a ritualistic display of passing (Scheper-Hughes, 1992). In addition, weddings, funerals and 'naming ceremonies' are often rich in religious narrative. Often all of the above include a gathering, big or small, in celebration of hopeful futures, whether that is in this life, in the case of a wedding, or in an afterlife, or celebration of life, as in the case of a funeral, wake and other burial ceremonies. I might also attempt to understand suffering culturally; for example, not all babies survive childbirth (Scheper-Hughes, 1992). Rites of passage ceremonies such as couples' union ceremonies, birth and death celebrations and such like, look to the future with hope because actually the future is unknown. If in the face of death, loss or tragedy, certain cultures, families or individuals turn to 'irrational' means as a way to make peace, even for a short while, then surely this means that hope lives on in a way that keeps the human condition alive. Hope-full and care-full spaces, realistic or not, are important in maintaining a 'good enough' life. How might we then incorporate this into a care ethics model of disability? As it is, Smith and Sparkes (2005: 1096), in their research on spinal cord injury, found restitution, transcendence, and chaotic narratives of hope. In reading their work on the restitution narratives I am prompted to think about the spiritual or faith. Their participants, the 'permanently' injured men designated as having a restitution narrative believed 'yesterday I was able-bodied, today I'm disabled, but tomorrow I'll be able-bodied again'. Similarly, within mothering narratives around intellectually disabled children one might say 'yesterday I was disappointed, today I suffer but tomorrow I will remain alive'. Of course this is not quite the same, but within the realms of believing or hoping that the suffering is temporary, such thoughts enable a mother to move through difficult moments and suffering, and therefore not be moved to take her life or the life of her child. This ability to engage with and believe in a hopeful future is important to bear in mind, as, for example, in Smith and Sparkes's research (2005: 1097), where Richard stated, 20 years after his injury, '[m]y hope ever since being in rehabilitation is that a cure will be found and I'll walk again'.

Belief and hope are crucial to survival. Hope and belief is the same for mothers living with an intellectually disabled child. Importantly it is within a Kantian interpretation of thinking about hope that three questions are posed: 'What can we know? What must we do? What may we hope?' (Ricoeur, 1995: 211) In an interpretation of Ricoeur it is crucial that the interplay between knowing, doing and hoping is respected as '[k]nowledge is what we can, doing is what we must, hoping is what we may, or are allowed to' (Ricoeur, 1995: 212). Scientific advances might give hope when there are rational answers, and of course it can be argued that we suffer less due to cures and new medical practices. Yet science is also dark, when it lurks over rights to life and whose life is worth living. Sometimes there are no answers, even temporarily, and to be left with a void without hope is too dark; hope gives life, in whatever form that takes. Significantly, taking into account Wilkinson's suffering, we can 'maintain that writing so as to involve readers in the great difficulty of understanding what suffering does to a person's humanity is an appropriate sociological response to this phenomena' (2005: 11). But as I said previously, hope is not enough; we must do, we must act, which is why a care ethics model must be enacted.

Tracy: an inhumane case

In drawing together suffering, hope and how I understand intellectual disability and mothering within a care ethics model of disability, I focus on a case from my previous research (Rogers, 2007a, 2013a). Here I highlight some thoughts with respect to living with disability and thinking about how inhumane – in a less 'extreme' sense than above – human beings are to each other. So, not literally life and death, but nevertheless quite care-less, unjust and systemically violent. Tracy is a white British, working-class mother in her 30s who has four boys aged between 11 and 16. Two of these children, the oldest, Dean (a twin), and the youngest, Brad, have (unrelated) different types of impairments. Both of her disabled children have been assessed for learning difficulties and received a statement of 'special educational needs'. I spoke to Tracy in detail about her experiences as a mother and how this has impacted upon her day-to-day life over the course of two in-depth interviews a year apart. Significantly, she has two very different disabling stories to tell, which seem largely dependent on the fact that even though Dean, her oldest son and a twin, drew on her resources as a carer in practical ways (although there were emotional responses too), Brad had additional behavioural difficulties that meant her care work, emotional labour and mothering identity were called into question, both by herself and by those around her. This is pertinent, as it is the difficult differences based on Brad's behaviours that, in part, produced the care-less space within which Tracy lived. Her other son, Dean's, mild physical and intellectual impairments were time consuming, but nevertheless not physically and emotionally exhausting in the same way.

Dean

Tracy's twins were born 29 weeks into her pregnancy and Dean's lungs collapsed immediately after birth. At five months old Dean was discharged from hospital, deaf, blind and paralysed. During this period Tracy travelled from East Anglia to London on a daily basis to visit him, even though she had his twin baby brother to care for at home. In the hospital Dean had probes attached to him which, if left too long in one place, made small round burn marks due to the low level of heat produced. She knew just this alone must have caused, at best, discomfort and at worst pain. It also had an impact on her relationships with 'early years' professionals, due to the fact that the marks left by the probes looked like old cigarette burns and Tracy was a smoker. In the early months seeing Dean lying in the hospital cot, Tracy told me 'I sometimes looked at him willing him to give up'. On leaving the hospital Dean had his first shunt put in – a piece of medical equipment for draining fluid from the brain for hydrocephalus. Tracy was very able to describe all the medical and technical aspects of caring for her son in a practical way. She told me she had watched the nurses for five months during his hospitalisation and had carried out her own research too (and she was a teenager at the time). This was the beginning of Tracy's caring story.

Clearly living with an intellectually disabled child can push a mother to question her love for her child, which often goes against culturally expected norms of loving your child unconditionally. However, Parker (1997: 17) refers to maternal ambivalence and sees this as a part of ordinary motherhood 'in which loving and hating feelings for children exist side by side'. Moreover, Moore (1996: 58) suggests that '[m]othering and motherhood are not, contrary to popular belief, the most natural things in the world', which is useful to keep in mind in contemplating the narratives discussed in this chapter. Listening to Tracy's story, it was clearly emotionally painful to see Dean in hospital with probes and monitors all over his body, not knowing if he would survive. At this point it could be argued that Tracy was existing within a care-full space, as institutionally and emotionally the caring spheres worked well for her, as she carried out her own practical care work on a daily basis.

Brad

Tracy's experience with her fourth son introduces a different caring story. She spoke to me of Brad's *different* behaviour from birth. She told me that as a baby 'he wouldn't give me eye contact or hold his head up', and that he 'had a cackle that was quite frightening'. She did go to the health visitors but nothing was noted as being problematic even though Tracy said that as a toddler 'he was very aggressive'. For example, with his brothers he would, she told me, 'walk up and kick them for no reason, pull their hair, bite them'. Given the cumulative, disruptive and aggressive nature of Brad's difficulties she did find her maternal self, emotional responses and caring roles at odds with each other. Tracy emphasised, 'I loved him to bits but there were certain bits that were wrong. I knew there were things wrong [...] But [...] (pause) I could never find the problem that existed'. Later on in the interview she was more graphic in her explanation of this love/hate dualism due to his disruptive and difficult behaviour. Tracy recalled that 'there were times when I'd sit there and I'd be like that gritting my teeth, (pause) I hated him, (pause) I loved him, but I hated him. I really detested him, the child he was, and what he did. I was in tears all the time'. This emotional dilemma and emotive language was based on aspects of her life that were dramatically affected, and as his mother she was expected to care for *and* care about Brad, unconditionally, to be continuously care-full. But what of caring when it involves, at best, disruption to the family as a whole and, at worst, emotional and physical pain for the mother? Based on this early caring encounter, we begin to see how care could be considered as maternal obligation and emotionally traumatic. It could be experienced as care-less. Although caring for, caring with, and caring about could be considered to be quite nebulous terms, how people interpret and experience them is an important issue for the one caring, the one caring with, the one cared for, policymakers, caring professionals and wider society.

Where practical care takes over: discussing Dean

Research suggests that a disabled child disables a whole family (Rogers, 2007b; Runswick-Cole, 2007). This is largely based on negative social perceptions of (and sometimes intolerance towards) disability (including difficult differences). As has already been evidenced, the social model of disability, whereby barriers to inclusion are considered socially constructed, was a reformative process for disabled people's experiences, particularly those with a physical impairment. This model translates into family research by suggesting that a disabled child disables the family based on social constructions of difference and disability leaking into and impacting upon family practices. The social model of disability was a reaction to many aspects of disablism, but also a response to the medical model which pathologised disabled individuals (see Oliver, 1996). These socially constructed barriers do have an impact on caring, as social intolerance leaks into daily life for mothers with disabled children and therefore limits experiences of carefulness and caring spaces. However, with regard to the everyday impacts of intellectual disabilities and for those experiencing 'impairment effects' (Thomas, 2007) (as experienced by mothers for example), the social model has not moved experiences and perceptions of disability and impairment as far forward as we might have anticipated (Oliver and Barnes, 2010; Shakespeare, 2006). Moreover, the social model falls short of addressing aspects of objective difficulties and emotional responses around impairments and behaviour considered to be outside culturally accepted norms, which are a day-to-day reality for some families. It is in response to this that a care ethics model that is based on interdependence and is relational is necessary. And it is this model that attempts to address systemic violence and inhumane acts that occur via the emotional, practical and socio-political caring spheres.

Thinking about caring and care-full-ness and what this might mean for a mother, especially in the early years, is often about practical necessity and actual dependence. As in Tracy's case, if the shunt for Dean's hydrocephalus was broken and not replaced the side effects could have been life threatening. Indeed, the very practical (day-to-day) aspects of caring work could also be considered as socio-political and emotional as the relations between these spheres is evident. For example, if something were to go wrong – the shunt breaks, Dean gets anxious about it, there are no caring professionals to hand, or there is no support for Tracy – all of these scenarios, while practically challenging for Tracy, are evidently emotional, and play into the hands of the socio-political (if no one is around to support Tracy the consequences could be life threatening). Even though Tracy had, as a mother, become a 'researcher' and a 'nurse', she was petrified at the thought of taking Dean home from hospital after watching the nurses for five months. But learning these nursing skills was crucial if she was to care for Dean competently. For example, he would stop breathing while taking his milk from a bottle. She told me, 'when I had friends round and we were watching tele and giving the baby the bottle [we] got wrapped up in conversation […] and [I'd] look down he'd be blue. […] he hadn't taken a breath'. She was told by the nurses what to do and pragmatically said that

> what you'd do is pull the bottle out and then we'd have to flick his toes and if that didn't work, pinch his toes and if that didn't work swing him round by his feet. Which sounds really weird [but] it was like second nature. I'd put me coffee down and off we go. Friends were quaking in their boots but it was just second nature coz I'd done it so often.

It is crucial for networks of friends to have some understanding of the caring involved, and it is here that the social model is not particularly helpful (especially in the private domain). For the first 18 months of his life Dean was visually and hearing impaired and paralysed, but Tracy said 'I absolutely adored him, but dreaded the future'.

Tracy emphasised that she was dreading him getting older and bigger and not being able to cope on a practical level. She also thought about how 'he would have no future, nothing to look forward to'. Tracy said she did have lots of family support and as a result often felt cared for and about, or as Lynch would argue, she experienced 'general care work' (Lynch, 2007) was done, but no one took Dean from her to give her a break as they said they were 'too frightened'. She went on, 'even though the doctors didn't hold out much hope, by the time he was two he could hear, see and sit up'. Extended early years caring often goes beyond what one would expect as a mother, and as a result can relate to absolute dependence, or at best interdependence. (Subsequently Dean went on to develop as a young adult and to gain some level of interdependence.) All of this, therefore, involved extended early years caring, both practically and emotionally. Dean was nearly 17 at the time of our first interview and Tracy said throughout that she wanted him to become self-sufficient and independent. Caring, both emotionally and practically, that goes beyond expectations of what mothering is on a day-to-day basis needs to be questioned. The narratives show how, sometimes, caring work (learning new skills to support a child) and caring emotionally (thinking and behaving with care) take over other day-to-day activities as the child develops. This day-to-day caring is often misunderstood, as in British policy, as partnership discourses suggest that there *is* support 'out there' (DfES, 2001a, 2001b, 2005, 2007; Rogers, 2011) for families with disabled children. Yet the battleground and the care-less spaces inhabited make caring work at times unbearable, and invoke suffering. The mother (in this case Tracy) might actually be carrying out caring work similar to that of paid care professionals (Hochschild, 1983; Theodosius, 2008). Crucially, though, this blurs into 'love labouring', according to Lynch (2007), due to the intimate relationship and lack of financial exchange, and, I would argue, the habitation of care-less spaces.

Carefullness, resilience, survival and skills development are evident in mothers with disabled children. However, once thoughts of survival (or not) in any immediate sense wane, the issue of the potential for lifelong caring is considered. This emotional lifelong caring, however, is not always associated with practical caring, but with 'love labouring' (Lynch, 2007). Of course there are indeed practical care issues with lifelong caring, but the idea of the future and the emotional responses to 'What next?' are crucial in the caring narrative. Living with their adult child's impairment and considering what that future holds are critical in ethical caring and care-full spaces. What is often missing from policy discourse and care professionals' training is the focus on the *family's* lifelong caring. Caring and care-full-ness ought to be privileged and positioned as not simply about the practical day-to-day aspects of caring (although these are important) but about how practical caring work and emotional work co-exist. Moreover, in addition to this, the mother who is caring for, about and with her 'child' faces potential prejudice, in addition to self-doubt about her own mothering abilities, as can be seen below.

Morality and humanity in mothering

I have so far discussed how the dark side of mothering manifests in response to other happenings that are sometimes outside of our control, like the death of a child, suffering and intense social pressure, and extreme caring. But if we remember the first set of quotes in the chapter, and particularly the one about wanting peace, mothering an intellectually disabled child can sometimes provoke feelings that go against what we consider to be 'normal' caring and loving feelings, to the point of not being able to cope, particularly if the child does not always act in a way that is perceived as socially acceptable. Yet also recall Sara's focus on wanting to recount the happy stuff in narrating her 'disabled' life. Janice McLaughlin and her colleagues suggest life with an intellectually disabled child is

> never boring, always lively, sometimes not the lively type that you would like and other times when it's absolutely hilarious, and other times you're just about pulling your hair out and just thinking I just cannot cope anymore, but you do, and you get up and get on with it.
>
> (McLaughlin et al., 2008: 102)

That fluctuation between loving a child and reflecting upon their sometimes difficult behaviour, though, can be emotionally draining and occasionally care-less, especially if it goes against culturally prescribed norms. Mothering a child whose actions call into question her caring, moral compass and maternal relationship is challenging.

The very essence of what it means to be a moral, care-full human being can go unnoticed, until the moment a mother's child acts in a way that is immoral, unethical and seemingly without responsibility. Connor, Sara's son, for example, was sectioned after he punched a teaching assistant (see Justice for LB, 2015b), and whilst this act is difficult to condone, it nevertheless needed to be dealt with in a care-*full* and caring manner. What happened after was wholly care-*less*. Several mothers interviewed as part of my research referred to difficult behaviour that *did* impact upon their caring and their emotional responses to aspects of their definitions of moral, ethical and responsible actions (Rogers, 2007a). They even questioned the humanity of their own child in the context of what it is to be a 'normal' caring and ethical human being. In my research, this difficult and challenging behaviour included public masturbation, self-induced vomiting, boys touching girls inappropriately, and criminal damage. Sometimes mothering and mothers' caring work veered between a duty of care (or obligation) and love/hate responses that questioned their maternal identity and actual *desire* to be caring and care-full. To draw on Tracy's story a little more, she had different experiences with each of her sons. She talked to me in her interviews about how Dean's behaviour towards girls younger than himself was problematic for her as a woman and as his mother, and about Brad's behaviour that was so verbally and physically violent that she feared for his or others' lives.

Ultimately Tracy felt responsible for their behaviour. With Dean, Tracy said

> (there were) possible sexual undertones with the younger girls, but I think what his body was saying 'hey I've got lots of hormones' (pause) this was when he was about 14, 15 and 'I've got lots of hormones here I'm a man' but mentally he relates better to smaller children because of his mental age, and he made friends with a little girl [...] and he used to play with her

and tickle her and (pause) although nobody ever said that he'd touched her sexually (pause) because of his size, and looking like a full grown man (it was) inappropriate for him to be playing with a 7, 8 year old girl.

This aspect of sexual behaviour was also introduced by other mothers in my research (Rogers, 2007a). What Tracy said about Dean's difficult behaviour and his intellectual capacity to understand his actions did cause her to contemplate her capacity to behave in a caring manner, partially due to how she felt about this inappropriate behaviour. Critically, Tracy's caring and carefulness here goes beyond Dean as it involves care for others, in this case anyone Dean touched inappropriately.

To introduce Brad into this narrative, and Tracy's caring in his case, she said, 'by the time he went to primary school, parents were complaining about him […] I was embarrassed because he was totally disrupting a whole class', but this was nothing compared to the disruption on a grander scale, as she described here:

> One day when he was 6 I was driving past the school and I saw some guys I knew who were installing windows and I stopped to chat to them and they said 'oh bloody hell, there were some fire engines up here earlier' […] And they said 'I bet your Brad set fire to the school', and I said 'yeah right' and we were having a right laugh about it (pause) and lo and behold when I went to collect him from school that night I got called into the school and he'd burnt down 2 portacabins [temporary buildings] and their contents! (She exclaimed).

As a result of this behaviour Brad was permanently excluded from school, which impacted not only upon Tracy's emotional response to the situation and how she felt, but also on her caring work, as he was not placed in another school immediately. She also told me she was subjected to aggression and hostility from parents who were worried about their own children being around such a 'dangerous and disruptive child'. This was a care-less space in every way. Consequently, due to the nature of Brad's behaviour he was tested and found to have a rare chromosomal syndrome that – according to medical professionals – meant he was more likely to display aggressive behaviour. Tracy at this time said that she felt vindicated as she knew all along that there was 'a problem with Brad' and not with her as a mother.

The incident above was not the only extreme behaviour displayed. Tracy explained that Brad had 'lit the gas fire and shoved the newspaper in the grill', and went on to say that he had 'stolen money from school out of teachers' handbags, police have been involved where he's threatened other children with a knife'. In fact a whole host of events over a period of a few years had happened involving both Tracy's actual day-to-day caring work and all spheres of the emotional, practical and socio-political caring spheres. Graphically Tracy told me 'we've had three portable teles (televisions) thrown from upstairs windows. [...] I've had neighbours knocking on my door saying "Brad's hanging out the window" [...] hanging by his fingertips'. Tracy struggled with a lack of support in this case and told me

> I used to have a really good babysitter for the other three children [...] but once Brad got a little bit older she was sitting in the chair like that and he came up behind her and held a knife at her throat and said 'I'm going to fucking kill you' and she wouldn't step foot inside the house again. Erm (pause) he's thrown knives at me, he's thrown knives at his brothers erm (pause) at this point the social services were a complete waste of space.

Essentially Tracy was in a care-less space, and it could be suggested that 'general care labour' (Lynch, 2007) or care-full networks were not available to her at this time. In addition to the above, before Brad was excluded from school, Tracy had to be present on the school premises at every break time due to his difficult behaviour. This meant that Tracy could not take paid employment during this period. This care-less-ness within the socio-political sphere ought to be addressed via the care ethics model of disability.

Considering caring work and carelessness, Tracy mentioned on several occasions how she phoned up the local authority for professional support, and told me 'I said (to social services) "so basically I've got to kick the shit out of my child before you do anything?"' She was refused any caring at that time. Eventually Brad was accommodated in a residential school for children with 'challenging behaviour' where he was a weekly boarder. Tracy by that point was desperate for some respite. Even when she did receive some caring she said she wanted support and respite, not therapy. Tracy simply wanted and needed 'time out' to experience care-ful-ness, and as a result told me

> a couple of times I thought about taking the lot of them [pills] and a big bottle of booze and just finishing it all [...] I got to the stage where I thought I was a completely lousy mother and they'd be better off without me anyway [...] I was getting to the stage where they would be better off without me.

In getting to this point, that of, at the very least, considering taking her own life, we are brought back to the beginning of the chapter where mothers have actually taken their disabled child's life and attempted to take, or actually taken, their own too. The examples above highlight the complexity involved in dealing with the care-less-ness that leaks into and out of all caring spheres. Critically, it is here therefore that social intolerance and care-less-ness in their broadest conceptualisation need to be recognised as problematic, so that mothers are emotionally able to experience care-ful-ness.

For Tracy, emotional caring was so overwhelming that she told me, 'there comes a time when your energy is so low that it affects your emotional state'.

This caring work shifts beyond financial and practical caring into a more ethical debate about who cares and what this means for an individual's everyday caring experience. Crucially, relationships between families and professionals must not be about individualistic notions based on particular professionals, but indeed there should be a 'politics of recognition', and moreover, that that recognition is a 'central component of social justice' (McLaughlin et al., 2008: 190).

Care-full mothering: concluding remarks

Why have we got a mother on the edge and even thinking about suicide? Whether this is just a passing thought, a serious consideration, or an act that is carried out, we need to think about caring and care-full spaces and ethical and just practices for mothers with disabled children. This ought to be considered within the socio-political sphere, as a reaction against social intolerance and an instigator for a more humane, ethically caring and just social position. In this chapter it seems that sometimes a mother might love and hate her child at the same time, but feels obliged to care for her. A mother with a disabled child is obliged to care, one could argue. The constant battle between 'I must do something' (caring for) and 'something must be done' (caring about) is critical in attempting to understand a complicated relationship (Noddings, 1995: 11). 'I must' carries with it 'obligation' (Noddings, 1995: 11); 'I must' is very different to 'I want'. It could be argued that some of the maternal narratives are driven by 'I must' and others by 'I want'. A mother with an intellectually disabled child might ask 'Do I love my son who has damaged the rest of our family?' and 'Do *I* care for him'? 'Yes I care' we might say, 'but love? That is more difficult: I both love and hate him'. Can we consider this caring and care-full?

Furthermore, in discussing mothering, it is clear that there are gendered issues. Women, for example, who do not express their emotions in response to the grief of others or do not respond tenderly to a crying baby are considered, at best, selfish. This is not the case with men (Friedman, 1995: 64); but for some mothers in my research there are times when practical caring takes over from emotional caring. Fundamentally, '[i]f caring is to be maintained, clearly, the one – caring must be maintained' (Noddings, 1995: 26). This is certainly the case for mothers with intellectually disabled children. Noddings (1995) implies that natural caring is something that is maternal, but that ethical care is outside of this relationship. This is based on a Kantian interpretation that ethical caring is done out of duty and not out of love, which is an interesting and important point to make, especially as not all maternal caring acts we have seen here are based on what might be described as 'natural caring', but are perhaps more likely to be interpreted as 'ethical care' (Noddings, 1995).

Death by indifference and 'virtual' support, other people's responses to an intellectually disabled person, as well as the care-full support and care-less suffering experienced is evidenced in this chapter. And as a result of taking the three caring spheres into account, I build upon a care ethics model of disability via formal and informal education from the previous chapter through to mothering and caring here. As it is, we need the model from cradle to grave. I again draw upon an ethics of care, for example with Held (2006), Noddings (1995) and Tronto (1993), and love labouring (Lynch, 2007; Lynch, Baker and Lyons, 2009), as well as other sociological research, in discussing hugely emotive experiences and philosophical debates in not only the caring work that is carried out by mothers but what caring is given to them, emotionally, practically and socio-politically. I engage with suffering as it seems that suffering is a normal part of being human (Craib, 1994), but in extreme cases can be too much to bear, and inhumane (Cohen, 2001; Wilkinson, 2005). Still, it is in being human that we might be able to see a way forward from suffering. In this sense, then, we might consider *who cares?* As Noddings (1995) implies, natural caring is something that is maternal, but ethical care is outside of this relationship. Nonetheless, ethical caring is more nuanced than this. Care-full mothering indeed involves everyone. The following chapter takes us away from the maternal *per se,* although the mother and/or others caring play a part in all the caring spheres. Friendships and relationships are what make us human and, therefore, it is evident that understanding intimacy is important within the context of caring, a care ethics model and intellectual disability.

5   Sexual and friendship politics: considering relationships

Introduction

> Obscured by the limits of our own small worlds, we find it so very hard to grasp the plural worlds of others; and to recognize that although they are not quite the same as ours, we are surely all bound by a common humanity. We are blinded by the restriction of our little-minded parochialism, provincialisms, patriotism and patriarchalisms. Usually we do not even see this, let alone try to move beyond. And this is one sure pathway to the miseries of human social life: to its perpetual conflicts and, worse, to its human atrocities. We stigmatise, silence and ultimately slaughter those others who, in their millions, are not like us, those others who render vulnerable the safety of our world, those who become our enemies.
>
> (Plummer, 2015: 15)

Ken Plummer is writing within the context of cosmopolitan sexualities in this quote, but I consider this lens enlightening in discussing intimacy and intellectual disability, not least because those who are different to us are considered a danger or are in danger, and because

> [n]ormativity pervades our lives [...]. We not merely have desires: we claim that we and others ought to act on some of them, but not on others. We assume that what somebody believes or does may be judged reasonable or unreasonable, right or wrong, good or bad, that it is answerable to standards or norms.
>
> (O'Neill, 1996: xi)

We are condemned for behaviour that falls outside of what is culturally expected. Not being recognised as a potential sexual partner or experiencing lack of autonomy due to a physical disability (Sakellariou, 2012; Siebers, 2012), being socially and emotionally isolated as a result of mental illness (Gillespie-Sells, Hill and Robbins, 1998; Shakespeare, 2006) and feeling unloved, lonely and infantilised, as well as experiencing, at times, extreme governance and violence, because of an intellectual impairment (Desjardins, 2012; Hollomotz, 2011; Kelly, Crowley and Hamilton, 2009; Richards et al.,

2012) are all disabling and dehumanising. Yet while I might expect to see both care-full and caring spaces within this chapter as a result of intimacy and how caring relations are played out, often with emotion and in private, when it comes to sex, intimacy and intellectual disability, no matter how private it might seem, the socio-political sphere – where social intolerance and aversion to difficult differences are played out – will always interfere and leak into the emotional and practical spheres. Other people will continue to have a view on what is considered socially, legally and culturally appropriate, especially when it comes to the human body and relations. Many of us favour one cultural or religious discourse that defines what it means to do intimacy and anything that is outside of that is simply judged as wrong, disgusting, stigmatised and inhuman.

Sometimes intellectually disabled people do not understand the social or cultural context within which they live, and it is down to caring work and care-full relations to mediate such intimacies. Furthermore, intellectually disabled people do not inhabit one culture, country, ethnicity, sexuality or class, for example, yet they will always be interdependent and in relationships. The emotional, practical and socio-political caring spheres I have identified throughout this book offer ways into thinking through a care ethics model of disability, in understanding humanity and being human, when reflecting upon relationships, physical or not. For the purposes of considering sexual politics and intellectual disability, the emotional and moreover, psycho-social, lie at the heart of relations, the self and a care ethics model. It is here I wonder how the self exists in relation to another in particular circumstances and how a care ethics model of disability might support care-full relations. Are caring and care-full relations always about reciprocity, friendships and intimacy and how are they managed when evidently what we often consider as private feelings and actions are made public and are then interpreted by others? Intimacy and relationships for intellectually disabled people has been storied in a way that is beyond caring and friendship and is indeed care-less. Often described as unable, unwilling, too willing, uncaring, not worthy, intellectually disabled people have been left without care, lonely and dehumanised. I would like to identify how intimate relationships and friendships benefit the everyday and how they can positively promote care-fulness across all three caring spheres within a care ethics model of disability.

Humanity, friendship, and care-full work

Discourses and representations of, and commentaries about, intellectually disabled people and their sexual and intimate life are pervasive. As Kim (2011: 481) says, 'disability has been defined by "defect" and "disorder" that presuppose an anatomically standardized and normalized human body, certain functions, and specific aesthetics. Thus, disability depends on ideological, social, and medical categories that determine what constitutes as average body, ability, trait and performance'. Furthermore, sterilisation has been justified in the name of 'best interests', because '[t]he feeble-minded (sic) have no forethought and no self-restraint' (Ellis in Pfeiffer, 2006: 83). On a global scale, many people consume media images of intellectual disability and sexuality where social and sexual awkwardness, infantilisation, and vulnerability are portrayed. Therefore, despite research in the area of sexual, relationship and reproductive life for and with intellectually disabled adults (Hollomotz, 2011; McCarthy, 2009, 2010), we have some way to go in breaking down the negative imagery, misrepresentations and discourses surrounding intellectually disabled people and their sexual and intimate lives (Haller, 2010).

Arguably, there has not been enough work done in understanding relationships and the importance of friendships (intimate or otherwise) within intellectual disability research, although there is some mention of it in places (Hollomotz, 2011; Rogers with Tuckwell, in press; Shakespeare, 2006). However, we do know how important intimacy and friendship relations are generally in human interaction (Pahl, 2000; Smart, 2007; Spencer and Pahl, 2006). Furthermore, friendship has been a concern for centuries, as, for example, in de Montaigne's (1533–1592) work it is argued that '[f]riendship on the contrary is enjoyed in proportion to our desire: since it is a matter of the mind, with our souls being purified by practicing it, it can spring forth, be nourished and grow only when enjoyed' (1991: 6), and Foucault, in discussing Greek culture, reflected that '[i]f you look at Plato, reciprocity is very important in friendship' (Rabinow, 1984: 345). In a particular fashion, Gibran, who published *The Prophet* in 1923, has been popularised and widely quoted at relationship ceremonies emphasising love and friendship (amongst other things) as crucial elements in successfully being with others. He says about friends that '[y]our friend is your needs answered' (Gibran, 1996: 35).

While friendship narratives might seem a little trite, there are many writers across disciplines who talk about the need and desire for friendship (Spencer and Pahl, 2006). Also, unless our liberty to make and keep friendships is taken from us (as is the case, often, for intellectually disabled people), it can be difficult to recognise the importance of such human interactions. These understandings have more recently been discussed within intellectual disability research as Turner and Crane (in press) point out. For example, Milton, a man in his 50s who spoke of being alone, wanting friends and sometimes feeling sad about all of this, told them:

> I like to be friends with them and sometimes, uh, they don't want to be friends with me or, uh, socializing with me. And, uh, sometimes it makes me lonely at times. And, um, sad, but, I just go on, do my, just do what I want to do. And just be alone and stuff. [...] it's bad when I want, uh, when you don't have nobody to talk to.
>
> (Turner and Crane, in press, n.p.)

Milton was not alone in this, as Richard, a man in his 40s, said, '[u]m, like I, always get lonely and play my games. No one to talk to' (Turner and Crane, in press, n.p.). It is important, therefore, to understand the dehumanising impact of restrictions on friendships, or simply the lack of friendship interaction and reciprocity for intellectually disabled people in the emotional caring sphere.

Not only are intellectually disabled people often left wanting, but the desire to make and keep friends is highlighted further in the worrying trend of 'mate crime' (Cassidy, 2015, Hollomotz, 2011; Thomas, 2011, 2013). This is where many young people desire friendships but lack the capacity to recognise that these 'friends' are behaving in a bullying, abusive and/or violent manner. This is similar to how domestic violence is experienced and narrated according to Pam Thomas (2011: 110) as she says, 'The desire for a relationship of some sort, the grooming and the servitude bear many of the hallmarks of domestic violence. "Mate crime" is not always sexual partner violence'. Furthermore, Cassidy (2015) highlights examples where one young autistic man said 'I was frightened to tell anyone about the bullying and theft and manipulation', and a young man said of his autistic brother '[m]y brother was befriended by neighbours who robbed him and stored drugs in his flat' (Cassidy, 2015: para. 5). Here we see differing examples of evidence that there are care-less and dehumanising day-to-day experiences, within the emotional 'caring' sphere, but also within the legal (Criminal Justice System) and socio-political sphere. This needs addressing urgently. Furthermore, it was found that those most vulnerable to 'mate crime' were aged 16–25: 'Every respondent in that age group reported having difficulty distinguishing genuine friends from those who may bully or abuse the friendships in some way' (Cassidy, 2015: para. 9). Both Cassidy (2015) and Hollomotz (2011) found that so-called 'friends' were directly involved in manipulating intellectually disabled people into illegal activity, as above with the drugs. Moreover Hollomotz (2011: 110) identifies that one of her research participants, Britney, suffered threats because her so called 'friends' wanted her to 'store stolen goods' and she was reluctant. It is worth, in this context, revisiting the case of the teenage intellectually disabled girl who was sexually abused by a gang of peers that I highlighted in Chapter 1. As it is, when she recounted the horror to the police over time, she continually expressed that these abusers were her 'friends' (Lefkowitz, 1998), thereby emphasising the desire to be friends, to be liked, and to be around others, despite her abusive, violent and harrowing experiences.

I too have an understanding of such 'mate crime' as on many occasions over the years my daughter has talked about 'friends' who were clearly bullying her in one way or another. The way this abuse is carried out is pervasive, as not only is it via physical and verbal interaction, but it also, with the increase in social media, leaks into the home, the bedroom, and wherever a phone or computer is accessed. The private space, the emotional 'caring' sphere, becomes a care-less space. Notably, sociologists emphasise the potential changes in social networks and see friendships as impacting upon not only the emotional, but also the practical and the socio-political caring spheres, as '[f]riendship is sure to grow in social and political importance as traditional forms of social glue decline or are modified' (Pahl, 2000: 12). We can see this demonstrated in intimacy and family research, as different ways of reconstituting personal networks and 'family' based on choice rather than heritage grow in significance (Gabb, 2008; Smart, 2007; Smart and Neale, 1999). Yet, as acknowledged above, if friendships (over and above family, for example) become ever more important in everyday networks, maintaining and negotiating larger and more disparate geographical spaces is evermore disabling for intellectually disabled people. Largely because this 'choice' of close and personal ties is already fractured, and then without care-full networks, barriers to personal and intimate ties exist and persist. We all rely on those who care for, with and about us in many areas of life and ultimately would prefer to feel secure in the choices we make about close connections (see Robinson, 2011a). This area of intimacy, therefore, moves us into thinking about the practical, where I consider how sexuality and relationships are managed, enabled and cared for, but it is across all spheres that care-less spaces exist.

For many, the management of personal relations might go unnoticed, but for intellectually disabled people this can become part of practical caring work (in a professional capacity) and emotional caring work (mothering, friendships, family and others) (Hollomotz, 2011; Rogers, 2009a, 2013a; Shakespeare, 2006). Third parties, other people, become involved in what is generally considered a private and intimate matter, (how we negotiate friend-ships, whom we have sex with and so on), and the loss of agency is palpable. This public–private blurring is problematic and can be care-less and dehu-manising. I have certainly experienced being a reluctant third party in my own daughter's intimacy journey (Rogers, 2009a), as well as being a nego-tiator in leisure space as a key worker in previous employment for intellec-tually disabled adults. I still am a reluctant third party for my daughter as we negotiate place, space, and relations, and this is an ongoing mediation process for many intellectually disabled people in their interdependent relations. This is evident in Banks' (in press) research, where she identifies borders to, and governance of, relationships as challenging. Here she describes how Vic, a support worker, (research participant) who chaperones Ellie, a young intellectually disabled woman, on her dates, negotiates caring spaces, care-fully. Vic had to get more involved emotionally and practically than he would have liked, as Tim, Ellie's boyfriend, told Vic, when he went to pick him up, that he wanted to break up with Ellie. Vic had to relay this emotionally charged break up narrative to Ellie and then continue to go to the same restaurant as expected, but without Tim, her boyfriend. According to Banks (in press), this put Vic in an incredibly uncomfortable position and she writes:

> Vic was left unprepared for the situation [...]. The break-up, though, changed the role that Vic had to perform. No longer just a protective agent, patrolling the borders between Ellie and Tim and the rest of us, Vic's experience of this event drew attention to the tension at the heart of

his work: the conflict between supporting Ellie to lead a rich life, while policing the border that keeps us safe from any possible transgressions.

(Banks, in press, n.p.)

This is not an unusual occurrence in disability research where professional others (or mothers) are involved in intimate aspects of disabled people's lives, but this moral, as well as practical, dilemma does require further contemplation (Bowlby et al., 2010; Carlson and Kittay, 2010) as intellectually disabled people are either governed or left wanting.

In many ways this intrusion of caring support into the personal is the antithesis of what intimate relationships are about emotionally, nevertheless it is necessary in some cases. The blurred boundaries around caring for, about and with when it comes to intimate relations confuse sexuality and relationships for intellectually disabled people (Rogers, 2009a). Consequently the emotional, practical and socio-political caring spheres leak into and out of the sexual, relational and intimate lives of intellectually disabled people. The socio-political, as an all-encompassing care space, or rather care-less space, interrogates how cultural scripts feed dehumanising processes for intellectually disabled people around their relationship life. Subsequently, to understand sexual and relationship politics through the lens of violence, infantilisation and exclusion is critical. It is the infantilisation of intellectually disabled people, or indeed their dehumanisation, that aids systemic violence and exclusion within social, community and political life. It is at this point that people are governed, surveyed and denied sexuality, intimate relationships, friendships, reproductive rights, and often even control over their own bodies. However, as evidenced above, I call for a care ethics model that cuts across all spheres, otherwise intellectually disabled people will continue to be abused, violated, stigmatised and dehumanised.

Care-lessness embodied: where is the love? Friendships and intimacy

'That's it. I'm not letting any more of her blokes into our lives,' I shouted, shattered and angry. Understandably so, as it was gone midnight and we had just left the police station having had a (now ex) boyfriend of Sarah's verbally abuse me and attempt to hit me. I got away mind you, as I was far quicker than he, even though he wouldn't let me out of my car and was kicking it. I was cornered until my husband talked him round, albeit temporarily, and for a moment the boyfriend moved away from the back of the car. My husband jumped in and we screeched off like something from a movie. 'I don't think I can drive, I feel sick,' I screamed, my heart pounding. Still I didn't want to stop. This lad was not someone you would want to upset, as rationale in this sort of a mood was not part of his personality once provoked, and I had seen that temper simmer with his Nan on the receiving end. I certainly did not want this for Sarah, especially as I had recently found out she was texting an ex-boyfriend. Irrational jealousy was not pleasant under ordinary circumstances. 'It's all such a mess.' I broke down and cried. Sarah, my daughter, then 20 years old, was taken to her Nan and Granddad's in an inconsolable state and wanting to leave home, this was before we went to the police station. [...] 'This is just too much,' I continued, as we planned how Sarah and I would flee the house for a few weeks. 'I'm coming to your house and I'm going to kill you. I will be with Sarah till we die,' he had hollered as we speedily left the rough road. I was scared. We fled, and for that summer if she was not palmed off on accommodating family members, she remained a prisoner in her own home. Not least of all because of the danger this violent young man posed, who himself was learning disabled and had other emotional and behavioural difficulties. [...] 'All she wants is to love and be loved,' I sigh.

(Rogers, 2009a, 271–272)

This quote is from an auto ethnographic paper I wrote a few years ago, about a very challenging situation involving my daughter and an intellectually disabled man who had additional challenging behaviours. They were dating (platonically, as far as I know) at the time, but the situation quickly became abusive. This excerpt and circumstance starkly, pessimistically and brutally talks of how intimacy, friendship and desire can spiral out of control. It also vividly illustrates Plummer's (2015) sentiment described in the opening quote to the chapter, because if humanity fails to consider circumstances beyond the small parochial nature of one's lot – in this case a young woman, man and the families involved, the socio-political, emotional and practical caring spheres will never be anything more than care-less.

What the excerpt also illuminates is that 'Sarah' so desperately wanted to be loved and be in a relationship/intimate friendship that she would remain in an abusive one rather than be 'alone'. Yet this story about desire, violence and abuse could have been told by any number of women or men in challenging relationships. In essence, if you have no friends or lovers life can be bleak and care-less (Spencer and Pahl, 2006; Turner and Crane, in press). So what makes us human, and why consider the importance of intimacy and friendships (sexless or otherwise) within sexual discourse? If humanity were based purely on the physical then we would be animal rather than human, but we are social beings; reproduction and sex alone do not make us human. In being human we are relational and have some kind of interaction, contact and – in whatever form it takes – communication, and often community. Moreover, we need emotional connection.[1] This can be via care-full touch, talk, or any other sensual and caring interaction. This is because, as I have found, people often want to be with other people (Arendt, 1998; Stienstra and Ashcroft, 2010), and need to experience caring over their life course (Kittay, 2005; Lynch, Baker and Lyons, 2009). Indeed, carelessness is dehumanising; loneliness and emotional isolation are damaging to the essence of being human, to our mental and physical health (Pahl, 2000; Smart, 2007). So is physical and emotional abuse – always. This emotional, practical and socio-political caring lack has been evidenced over the decades, as individualism erodes humanity and caring spaces (Bauman, 2003, 2007; Lasch, 1991; Robinson, 2011a).

As research around intellectual disability and sexual rights, sexuality, genetics, reproduction and so on develop, the more nuanced and mundane aspects of day-to-day living, caring, loving and friendships for example, are not privileged. Rights to have sex, reproduce, rear a child, have control over one's body and so on are on the political agenda (Ledger et al., in press; Richards et al., 2012). Promoting friendship and caring might seem innocuous, and I do recognise it is challenging to legislate about caring and loving, although not, maybe, an impossible task. As '[o]ur legal structure would not be based on individualist models privileging autonomy and independence [...] Rather each person's need and rights would have to be considered in the context of their relationships' (Herring, 2013: 86). Critically, we can see, in friendship research, that these human relations are crucial for mental health. Indeed, with socio-political and community changes we need to consider these aspects of human life for intellectually disabled people as a matter of urgency. It is not just for the caring few but that 'internationally a caring world would be one in which the essential needs of citizens around the world would be met. We should be seeking not only caring individuals, but caring institutions and governments' (Herring, 2013: 87). Certainly, as changes over time have occurred, de-institutionalisation has taken place and community care projects have developed in the name of a broader care discourse, yet many 'disabled people are in the community, but not part of the community' (Shakespeare, 2006: 175).

Importantly, it is within a human relations narrative that so many intellectually disabled people position themselves when asked. In Hollomotz's (2011) research, losing friends or not having friends in the local community is a problem. This is often due to services and education provision being 'somewhere else' or changed without consultation. For example, 'Rose states that one of her friends attends a different day service venue since her day service was reorganised. She has not seen him since and she has no means of keeping in touch with him' (Hollomotz, 2011: 92). This is not an isolated case and, put simply, it is inhumane. How many people have friends taken, never to be seen again? Some may be taken in tragic circumstances, and then there is a grieving process to go through. People who are not intellectually impaired do not have this type of restriction imposed upon them. I can, of course, think of some other examples where friendships might have restrictions placed upon them due to religious, cultural or geographical barriers, and many of these cases might also be inhumane and care-less in removing friendship interaction. But processing this loss might be informed. For example, when people move location due to work or changing domestic circumstances they also move away from their friendship networks. However, most are able to maintain these friendships via social media or other such means. The same cannot necessarily be said for those with additional challenges and constraints such as an intellectual impairment and/or lack of access to social media. The transient nature of friendships is not one that is chosen for intellectually disabled people, nor is it even considered by many professional support staff or within broader socio-political directives. This systemic violence, where friend-ships and intimate relationships are deemed meaningless, mobile, transferable and inconsequential is abhorrent, love-less, unethical, care-less and inhumane.

In a small research project my intellectually disabled daughter and I carried out on sexuality and relationships, friendships were certainly a large part of the narrative, as indicated here and further on below in field notes from a focus group (Rogers with Tuckwell, in press):

> It was a bright yet cool day with the threat of rain. There were five intellectually disabled young people aged between 23–30 years; three women and two men, myself and some other researchers. The focus group took place in a large, bright, airy, echoey room of a church hall. I did all the usual pleasantries, ground rules and introductions. We were all there for the same reason: to consider friendships, intimacy and relationships.

They all went on to say how much they wanted friends. Yet this friendship narrative was not what we had planned at the outset of the study as the main questions were focused upon mapping how young intellectually disabled people make sense of their intimate, emotional and relationship experiences, exploring how parents (or carers) understand and engage with their intellec-tually disabled child's sexual identities and relationships, and mapping and recording how to do research inclusively (Rogers with Tuckwell, in press).

Despite the project, and therefore the focus group, being promoted as sexuality and relationships research, many of the narratives were about transport (to go to and from meeting with friends), money (to enable social activity), being with friends and boyfriends (or not spending enough time with them) and talking about the future (getting married, having a family and such like). The reasons behind this are identified here in our field notes below.

> The opening question was very broad, 'so why did you decide to get involved in this research?' Ben piped up 'I want to learn a lot from this experience, I really think I'm going to learn about friends and relation-ships, I also want to make new friends.' 'I want to make new friends too,' chipped in Teela 'especially female ones so that I can talk about things girls talk about.' 'I'd like to make more friends, but I also really want to spend more time with my boyfriend,' Kerry exclaimed. George agreed with the group saying he wanted to make new friends, but actually saw this group as a way also of getting to know those he knew already a little better.
>
> (Rogers with Tuckwell, in press, n.p.)

This excerpt indicates the enormity of a caring and social life, and on reflection I am reminded of what 'friendship' and social interaction can mean for particular groups of people, as I noted last year in my own personal reflections.

Sitting here with my iPad looking through my Facebook account and a picture of my daughter pops up. She is 27 years old. A beautiful head shot. A few likes on Facebook from family members and I do the same. But then what happens is a torrent of narratives that go on between two young women and my daughter's boyfriend of 4 and half years. There's lots of talk about how one young woman loves my daughter and the other girl agreeing, and my daughter's boyfriend is saying that this is not true. There are accusations of pictures of girls in underwear and all sorts. I know that my daughter doesn't really know this girl. This whole narrative exchange exceeded 200 comments! Why? Boredom? I can't really know. All I do know is that on talking to my daughter and her boyfriend they don't really seem to understand what it is all about. There is an element of naivety, but they are not young. Whatever – this interaction, this care-less moment was tricky for all concerned and did cause some upset.

(Personal reflections, 2014)

So looking at the focus group material and the above reflection, which involves relationships or the storying of relationships (whether true or not), we can see that sex is not always part of the narrative, although sometimes desire might be. I am not for one moment going to suggest sex and all the social justice and rights aspects that come with it are not important (especially when discussing marriage, reproduction and suchlike) (Ledger et al., in press; Richards et al., 2012), but in this discussion it is the relationship that is privileged within a discourse of caring and care-full relations.

As it is, people in caring relationships are, or ought to be, caring both for themselves and others (Held, 2006), but also it is important that '[f]riends can recognize each other as highly caring without constant demonstrations of care' (Held, 2006: 50). This is, as research has suggested, more difficult for intellectually disabled people, which is why it is even more crucial to understand friendships and intimacy within a broad care ethics model of disability. All people ought to be caring and care-full, not simply those who are family members or care work professionals with intellectually disabled people. Notably, Shakespeare has interrogated sexuality work and re-evaluated it in light of the broader friendship and intimacy research, and reminds us that

[a] century ago, we would have been socially and culturally determined by our family. Fifty years ago, this role would have been played out by our work and career. Now it is the people we do things with that count. Developing rich and varied social connections and having friends is a hidden but vital dimension of society.

(Shakespeare, 2006: 170)

This again highlights the importance of all of our relationships. He also draws on the work of Ray Pahl, suggesting that humans not only need to access material resources but also psychological ones so as to be fully involved in society.

Significantly, if you are not intellectually disabled but experience loss of mobility or 'free will' or have a near death experience, friendships, social support and intimacy are all emphasised. Notably, Pahl (2000) draws attention to this in a case where a British television presenter had a serious road accident, but then seven months later reflects upon her near death experience, and despite recognising the cliché says, 'I now consider friends and family to be far more important' (Pahl, 2000: 141) than work. Intellectually disabled people do not necessarily have the 'option' to reflect, choose and consider life paths relating to work, community and social networks in this way. Indeed, it is all too easy for non-disabled people to take for granted their own friendship and support networks, as '[e]ven where disabled people have friends and companions, they may find it harder to experience everyday intimacies' (Shakespeare, 2006: 173; see also Lawson, 2005; McCarthy, 1999), which is compounded by young people's imagined futures that involve long-term relationships and children (Henderson et al., 2007).

Private acts, public scripts: bounded and boundary work

Let us consider making friends and becoming part of a social network and community. It is evident that many intellectually disabled people are already at a disadvantage due to emotional, practical and socio-political caring spheres (or care-less spaces). Despite the closure of large institutions, various supported living arrangements necessarily occur, particularly for those who are severely and profoundly intellectually disabled. This means that the private and public life of friendships and relationships are blurred. It is assumed that people's intimate and sexual lives are a private affair. However, sexuality is not simply a private matter or that of personal choice, and 'personal lives are never outside the discursive structures of society' (Carabine, 2004: 124). Besides, intimate relationships are often only surveyed in the public sphere when sexuality and sexual activity are deemed problematic, dangerous or risky, which is often the case when discussing intellectual disability. This might be due to abuse, vulnerability, threat of danger and so on. Significantly, some intellectually disabled people are confused about the staff/friendship relationship, and with good reason (Banks, in press; Feely, in press; Fish, in press; Hollomotz, 2011; Rogers, 2009a). This is largely because social workers, support workers and other 'care' professionals have designated clients to work with. They might sleep overnight in a staff bedroom, have a key to the front door, and do practical and emotional day-to-day work, including going out for social events and liaising with family members.

In thinking about boundaries and bounded work, I would like to revisit Banks' (in press) research in a little more detail. She writes about this aspect of bounded and boundary caring work and particularly focuses on one care-full working relationship. Her paper is drawn from a much larger project in an Australian city. As I have already identified, it is about Vic, a support worker, and focuses upon one momentous incident that he had to deal with – a relationship break up. Vic's usual responsibility as a professional care worker was that of 'taxi driver', or protector of/protector from perceived risk, as he mediated a relationship between Ellie and Tim, two intellectually disabled adults. He would drive Ellie to Tim's and then on to a café/restaurant/cinema. He would sit apart from them, and, as Banks puts it, act as a border control agent, limiting bad happenings. Yet he too is bounded and has boundaries. However, one night everything changed, as discovered above. Vic went to pick Tim up but Tim no longer wanted to see Ellie and shut the door; that was that. Vic's minor role in the story as mediator/facilitator turned into him becoming one of the main characters. He was thrown into feeling and recognising the pain, and sometimes discomfort, of being disabled. What many experience as a private affair (a break up) was public; it did not happen between just two individuals. In addition to that, Vic was no longer a surveyor, he was part of the surveyed, largely because he ended up dining out with Ellie, who was very obviously emotional, and others looked on.

These fractured boundaries between the private and public understandings of relationships can be acknowledged within my research as well as my personal experiences. Vic as a support worker did not expect Ellie and Tim's relationship to end, and certainly did not expect to get emotionally involved. My own previous position as a residential social worker illustrates how intimate friendships and relationships are difficult to negotiate and comprehend for some intellectually disabled people. This excerpt is taken from my auto ethnographic research (Rogers, 2009: 276–277) and I use it here for the purposes of engaging in a discussion about private and public boundaries and bounded work. In addition, it is useful to reflect upon the emotional and practical bond (or ties) between paid 'carers' and their clients, and the care-full and care-less spaces inhabited, both for professionals and for intellectually disabled people.

> I drove up the motorway on my way to work [...]. The sun was shining and all was pretty good. My role? A support worker for a charitable housing association and I often had sole responsibility for overseeing the lives of five learning disabled adults in their home. I did move around to other houses but the one I was heading to was my main place of work. 'Hiya Sam,' I called out as I came through the door with my own front door key. My colleague and I exchanged pleasantries and swiftly finished the handover procedure. This was particularly the case at the weekend. I spent the afternoon chatting to the residents, after which Sam and I started to sort out dinner. I had been working at this particular place for some time and Sam (a middle-aged black Afro-Caribbean man) was assigned to me. I was his key worker. Before he came to the house I had visited him in the mental health institution, spoke to him about the move to his new home and basically befriended him. He was on medication for violent behaviour, which seemed to make him docile and he rarely spoke. Sam came to the UK from the West Indies after a natural disaster. He lost his immediate family and his only other traceable family members

were in East London. Clearly distressed and with some learning difficulties and almost no speech, he was institutionalised for his erratic and violent behaviour and presumed mental health problems. As his key worker I had to set up a care plan, go shopping with him, visit places of leisure, support him in his chores around the house, prompt him on personal care issues and ensure he took his medication. Eventually as a team we decided to recommend his concoction of drugs were reduced in an attempt to alleviate his docility. As a support worker I would sleep overnight a couple of times a week and spend at least four or five days a week in and around the house. It was my place of WORK (my public environment), it was his place to LIVE (his 'private' environment). This private/public issue is important regarding both discussions about disabled people and sexuality. Not least of all because I was in effect an 'intruder' in Sam's house. But, I had my own key to his front door, and I became a 'friend'. [...] In Sam's case he certainly grew to consider me a friend (or even more). A year or so since Sam had arrived at the house and back to the afternoon in question, our relationship changed forever. I was alone in the house, (not unusually so) and in the kitchen with Sam. The six-foot man grabbed the waistband of my trousers, clear in his intention to undress me. I flung my hands in the air and shouted 'NO!' Shaken, I told him that was not my understanding of our 'relationship'. He did not pursue it and seemed genuinely upset by the rejection. I went to the 'sleep-in' bedroom, locked the door and rang my senior. 'Mary, there's been an incident,' I nervously said. 'Well, would you like to leave? Only you know you can't until someone else comes, but I can try to arrange cover.' 'No,' came my reply. I decided to stay, but remained in the bedroom with the door locked for the night. That night I lay in bed thinking about what had happened. What mis-understandings had occurred? I realised that Sam had read our relationship as something totally different. Thoughts span around my head as I tried to work out what had gone on. From my thoughts of past moments and in the small sleep-in bedroom I checked the door to make sure it was locked. 'Why would he not think that we were courting in some traditional way?' I mused. I was in his private environment. Out of all the staff I was his key worker, I was the one who went out with him, went to lunch with him and supported him. I genuinely cared about his life and what he did. Of course other staff members would play a part in his life but not in the same way I did. They were peripheral as I was with some of the other residents in the house. After a disturbed night's sleep I left the house the next day. [...] Sometime later and remembering, Sam withdrew from me and our relationship became more difficult. He was less accommodating. I tried to talk about it to him as did other staff members, but it seemed like a 'break-up'. All the staff at the house had known that there had been a couple of complaints filed against Sam for inappropriately touching women on the bus. I was concerned that if Sam thought he and I no longer had a 'relationship' that this type of behaviour would escalate.

This lengthy scene is important in describing friendship and relationship activity, but it also reinforces the notion that sexual desire based on the development of a caring and care-full relationship can inhabit boundaries, but can also be bounded. I was bound to my work, to Sam, to my caring role, yet there were boundaries that Sam and I interpreted differently. Deliberating over this particular example, it seems clear as to why Sam would think he and I were in a relationship. It was our own interpretations of the relationship that differed. As an intellectually disabled man he had no close friends and did not speak to anyone – not even those he shared a home with. As a full-time member of staff I was the closest person to him, in his life, on a day-to-day basis. As I say, I cooked, cleaned and slept overnight. When I rejected his physical advances after a year of 'being together', he understandably withdrew emotionally and practically.

This blurring of the intimate and private boundaries with the professional and public is not unusual for intellectually disabled people, particularly in the case of more violent and abusive relationships, as in the case of 'mate' crime (Thomas, 2011, 2013, Cassidy, 2015). At one level, for example, private acts are often mediated, or dealt with by professional caring others (or mothers). In my interviews with parents, Francis, who has a 12-year-old disabled son, talked openly about how he would behave inappropriately at home and in public. She told me her son was 'self-mutilating (sighs) forever masturbating and smearing faeces round his room, vomiting, he used to make himself vomit that was all round his bed and on the floor' (Rogers, 2007a: 75). As I have suggested, whilst not necessarily the norm, this is not an isolated case of sex-related behaviour, where parents and especially mothers or professional care workers have to deal with difficult and emotionally and practically messy situations. Their mothering (or caring work) crosses boundaries into seemingly more care-full work, we hope. These blurred private/public boundaries of sexuality and intimacy were evident in my workplace, where, for example, elderly parents would comment on whether their son/daughter was 'allowed' to have an intimate partner, and professional care workers would walk in and out of residents' bedrooms where it seemed no privacy laws applied (see also Fish, in press; Hollomotz, 2011).

Much recent research suggests that little has changed in the past decade, as Hollomotz (2011: 159) describes how 'staff would at times walk into a person's room without knocking' and relationships with staff 'were at times imbalanced and insufficient respect was given to other personal relationships that were of importance to a person' (2011: 159). Significantly, Shakespeare found that 'people with learning difficulties are isolated in subgroups of professional workers, and peers with learning difficulties' (Shakespeare, 2006: 172) where they struggle to develop caring networks. I too have found that more often than not, in my research, in my previous career and in my personal life, intellectually disabled people sometimes develop friendships with their support workers, or at least consider them a friend. But then, as I highlighted above, wanting friends, but maintaining caring and care-full friendships is not easy.

Even in the case of Sam in my work place, the relationship at a deeper level was always one-sided. Clearly this chapter has identified that friendship and relationships are critical for intellectually disabled people. But how does the socio-political sphere respond, react and create care-less spaces, where so much that happens beyond the personal, and where the negotiation of boundaries and psycho-social responses to cultural norms, leak into and out of day-to-day life? I propose that this occurs via the media and in the storying and representations of intellectual disability. I have already acknowledged the significance of representations of intellectual disability in Chapter 1, but identify here, in more detail, and with reference to intimacy purposively. This is because much of what we know, or think we know about differences, is played out on our screens, via the internet, through the news media and in film and television shows. This impacts upon understanding and interpretation of intellectual disability and is often a care-less space.

Fiction or fact: representing intellectual disability in care-less spaces

Through fiction and 'factual' representation, via the characters of Dopey in Walt Disney's *Snow White* and Tom Hanks' characterisation of Forrest in *Forrest Gump*; Channel 4's reality television show *The Undateables*; soap storylines (serial drama) via Sam Dingle in *Emmerdale*, Billy Mitchell in *EastEnders*; and Derek, the main character in Channel 4's mockumentary series *Derek*, we see, feel and interact with characters who we might want to love, look after, feel sorry for, and sometimes laugh at or with. Thus, Dopey in *Snow White* is different from the other 'dwarfs'. He looks different, is out of kilter, is clumsy and gets into trouble inadvertently, as well as being infantilised (Schwartz, Lutfiyya and Hansen, 2013). Dopey is 'not part of the group, always the last one to do anything, except when it came to undesirable things' (Schwartz, Lutfiyya and Hansen, 2013: 179). This film, aimed at children, tells a particular story about disadvantage and being marginal. As we view, interact and make meaning, social and cultural messages are learned: we find that some people are different from us (Berger, 1972; Hall, Evans and Nixon, 2013). But then in immersing ourselves we can both laugh at, and create a distance from, those who seem to be not quite human. For example, Billy Mitchell in *EastEnders* is considered a little 'slow' by his fellow characters, and as a result, like Dopey, always in trouble, is used to perform tasks that others would rather not carry out, and is more often than not considered in the community as unable to fully deal with his affairs. Similarly, Sam Dingle in *Emmerdale* is characterised as someone with a mild intellectual disability. He is a man in his 30s living at home with his family, but is, like Dopey and Billy, infantilised despite being employed and a father. He is often the butt of jokes, does not always get nuances about everyday life and unwittingly gets into trouble. Also, Sam does not always read social cues appropriately, especially when it comes to romance (like with the real characters in Channel 4's

The Undateables, as discussed below). This inability to read social cues, getting into trouble and so on, plays to the amusement of the audience and has reoccurred in storylines over the years. Moreover, much of what we see and imagine in these storylines has been played out in the research identified above.

Sam's storyline in 2014, in thinking about these friendship and relationship issues, had a more sinister edge to it. Sam began phoning an erotic chat line and 'befriended' a young woman called Tracy. He started to take money from the family funds to finance the expensive conversations. The implication in this storyline was that the chats were not sexual, which feeds into narratives around sexuality, or rather asexuality, and intellectual disability, or the understanding that Sam wanted a 'friend' rather than sexual pleasure. As the storyline progresses Tracy comes to Sam's home, gains a roof over her head and begins to manipulate Sam into buying her drinks, clothes and jewellery. He is duped into getting a credit card, and it is assumed by others that they are dating. As far as the audience could tell they had not had a physical relationship at that point. It is also obvious to the audience that he is being fooled, thus representing and reaffirming the naivety of people in our own communities like Sam. As with Dopey, the audience would not want to see harm come to Sam, and yet they can also distance themselves from him as 'Other', as 'not like us'. These narratives remind us of the real life desire for friendship and intimacy, and the potential abuse or 'mate crime' which may follow, as discussed above. What comes first, the image making, or the desire and abuse? *Emmerdale* is watched by millions, and, regardless of the classed nature of viewing soaps, it is the everyday element in talking about this to our neighbours, on the sofa, at work, that imagining, narrating and then Othering is part of how we see those who might not be considered fully human (just as discussed in Chapter 1, with the block busting shows). These storylines can either evoke pity or relief, where the audience sympathises with the character or feels relief that this is not their life.

In Channel 4's mockumentary series, Ricky Gervais characterises a middle-aged man named Derek who is intellectually disabled[2] and is the main narrator of a show about an elderly care home. As with Sam, Derek is a lovable character. He is a helper who befriends the elderly people who live there, but clearly he is childlike and innocent in how he sees the world around him. There are storylines, similar to those discussed above, where he struggles to date, is the butt of jokes and so on. Yet, I would argue, he is portrayed as having more humanity than any of those around him (except perhaps for the female lead). The good/evil binary that is often at play within disability narratives is evident here. He is everything that is good about the human being. He is characterised as stereotypical of an intellectually disabled person assumed to be in need of care and yet is beyond malice, not like some of the other characters around him who are generally mean. This provokes the viewer into thinking he is lovable, and possibly above humanity, because he simply sees the best in people, again representative of research in the previous chapter. His lack of human flaws (greed and lust, for example, which plague other main characters) make him seem angelic, not like the non-disabled viewer. Similarly to Derek, Sam and Dopey, the young intellectually disabled people in Channel 4's reality show *The Undateables* are positioned as innocent or infantilised. They are on the hunt for love, and in most cases they are portrayed, through no fault of their own, as unable to find an intimate companion. It is through the setting up of dates via dating websites and matchmaking that the film makers produce stories that draw the viewer in. But, importantly here, what we catch a glimpse of, via the narratives of the young people and in the edit, is that some intellectually disabled people have potentially unrealistic expectations of love, romance and life ever after. What the audience also participate in, as voyeurs, is the awkwardness and discomfort of intimacy. Silences, and a sometimes thwarted ability to interact with another human being comfortably, are both implicitly and explicitly projected throughout, just as with Sam in *Emmerdale*, and Ellie with Vic in Banks' (in press) research. Dis-ease, pity and embarrassment is what is experienced by the voyeur as the 'Undateables' do relationships.

We, as the audience, are invited into bedrooms that we would recognise as a child's, and we listen to young people's wildly ambitious expectations of marriage within hours of meeting their companion. Therefore the audience is left to decode these narratives and ultimately is given licence to assume that the relationship life for those who are intellectually impaired is unmanageable, sometimes asexual, infantile and therefore unrealistic in many cases. As the viewer we might want it to work, as with a fictionalised happy-ever-after story, but in most cases on the show it does not. In truth, however, as we understand from research highlighted throughout, many do not really want intellectually disabled people to have a sex life or to have children. In the cases discussed above, the image, meaning-making and interaction between the viewer and the viewed rely on cultural assumptions and norms about what we can expect, whether that assumption is based on falling in love, nurturing, friendships, intimacy, having a family, or something else. What all of these 'characters' lack, one might argue, is rationality. For centuries, and certainly since the Enlightenment, being fully human relies on reason and rationality, and there is most certainly a hierarchy (Davis, 2006; Schwartz, Lutfiyya and Hansen, 2013; Yar and Rafter, 2013), with those who lack reason at the bottom of the pile, or disabled others ending up in the 'dustbin' (Shakespeare, 1994). Indeed, the role images play in influencing our cultural narratives, social psyche and assumptions about intellectual disability are pervasive and begin from a very young age via characters in children's literature and film (Beckett et al., 2010).

While these images, cultural scripts and stories might seem playful and benign, children begin, through these, to understand the implicit, and sometimes explicit, messages about labels, stereotypes and stigma. I am not suggesting that viewers are unable to decode and see prejudice and suchlike as problematic, but many of the storylines are not explicit and so the underlying meaning for many intellectually disabled people is insidious. These storylines and characters have an impact not dissimilar to a very small tear in a pipe. The drip, drip,

drip of imagery about intellectually disabled people and their relationships seeps into the psycho-social, impacting upon our ways of being and thinking, our collective conscience, and then into the socio-political – they always have. Notably, Goffman (1990: 140), writing about stigmatised people, suggests that '[t]he individual is advised to see himself as a fully human being like anyone else, one who at worst happens to be excluded from what is, in the last analysis, merely one area of social life. He is not a type or category, but a human being'. Yet for intellectually disabled people it is not often as easy as taking on this mantle and 'seeing' themselves in this way. Their intellectual capacity to reflect in this way sometimes creates too many challenges. I have gone into some detail about friendships, but what about beyond this, moving into the realms of intimacy, sex and all that comes with it?

Sex and care-less spaces

Intellectually disabled people have 'distressingly been deprived of their sexual rights and, more specifically have been thought to be incompetent in their roles as sexual beings' (Richards et al., 2012: 103). The United Nations Convention on the Rights of Person with Disabilities and other legislative bodies say that intellectually disabled people hold these rights, and yet we know they are continually and systemically denied social justice within any kind of caring space. Currently, 'little progress regarding the sexual rights for people with intellectual disabilities has been achieved' (Richards et al., 2012: 103). Richards and her colleagues interrogate the United Nations rights discourse alongside real-life narratives from Barb and Murray, two intellectually disabled adults who only ever wanted to be together. While changes occur, it is abundantly clear that the socio-political caring sphere is indeed care-less and not yet doing enough to shift the legal and rights aspects of sexuality for intellectually disabled people. But crucially, too, the psycho-social – the emotional space where unknown others make decisions about the private sexual and reproductive life of those who may be unable to have what they want from life, which is more often than not a family, a lover and a friend – is left without caring, is care-less. This is de-humanising.

This aspect of desire and want is highlighted in Hollomotz's (2011: 63) research as Tyler, an intellectually disabled man in his 20s, tells her he wishes 'nothing more than a long term relationship' and says,

> I wanna be a dad ... I've always had this dream. I'm sat on the settee with my girlfriend in my arm and my child playing at the table and I'm watching television ... and I wake up with a smile on my face and a very warm feeling. I go: 'that's what I want'.
>
> (Hollomotz, 2011: 63)

Within a similar discourse, hoping for and planning a wedding and family is underlined in a personal vignette narrated by my intellectually disabled daughter with my support. It captures the everyday aspects of desire that many other young people dream of, or expect:

> Today is like any other day for Mum (out of term time). She had a cup of tea and cereal, helped me wash my hair in the bath and began to think about what writing she had to do. She wandered into the living room, and my pile of cut outs and Argos books are stacked up on my sofa. A note book open at a page with copied words. Mum shouts up the stairs, 'Sherrie can we throw out the old Argos book and some of these scraps?' The terror in my voice can be heard as I run down the stairs screaming 'NO!' 'But they are old and an unsightly mess. Please just some of it then,' Mum pleads. But no, not today – not ever.

My daughter and I, more recently, in a research meeting contemplate the seemingly innocuous and everyday characteristic of this conversation. But only on reflection, as nothing has changed. What lies beneath this particular story? Why is the Argos book so desperately important? At the time my daughter cut out pictures from a book every day. We discuss this again. What are these pictures of? Funky kettles and toasters, white goods, cots, beds, wardrobes and suchlike cover the pages of her scrap book. She also cut out pictures of wedding rings, engagement rings and other wedding related para-phernalia. As it happens, in the UK, traditionally some of these items might have been called 'bottom drawer items' (goods that a young woman collected for her married life). Critically here, though, for many young people, espe-cially those in supported living, the significance of taking away those 'scraps' can have a damaging emotional impact (see Hollomotz, 2011), yet many care professionals do not consider these 'scraps' as personal and important belongings as they tidy up around them. They do not consider imagined or real futures (see Hollomotz, 2011). Furthermore, my daughter's desire for and expectation of what she wants in life, as well as the desire of others in research more broadly, is clear. While there are many aspects to discuss, what I want to consider is the emotional interaction, being with people, and being cared for and about, as for intellectually disabled people, human interaction, the emotional connection and the everyday aspect of being with people are less secure (see Kittay and Carlson, 2010; Robinson, 2011a).

Simply, many moderately and profoundly intellectually disabled people do not have the same opportunities to meet people at work and socially. One of the contentious issues for intellectually disabled people is that due to their intellectual impairment they are infantilised, or assumed to be less than human, on the basis of their perceived and actual vulnerabilities (Hollomotz, 2011), their best interests (MCA, 2005), cultural perceptions, and fear (about the potential reproduction of more intellectually disabled people). All of this directly impacts upon their maintaining or losing intimate and friendship relations. Thus, to have a physical sexual relationship with another, one has to meet people: obvious as this is, it is a fact. Also, in many parts of the Western world, age and consent are a significant factor. Ultimately intellectually disabled people, due to their intellectual impairment, are legally, social and culturally infantilised. This is care-less and de-humanising. In the case of intellectually disabled women, they are often discouraged from getting married, having intimate relationships or reproducing (Hollomotz, 2011), and more often than not are also excluded from sex education due to an actual intellectual impairment and social immaturity, but more importantly because social perceptions and expectations of them preclude their inclusion. The transition to adulthood, unlike that of many young people, is in all aspects complex, and particularly in the development of intimate and sexual relationships and childrearing. At its worst intellectually disabled people are restricted in their sexual, intimate and reproductive activity (Ledger et al., in press).

Controversially, attention has been drawn towards intellectually disabled young people and their sexual activity or sexuality, which has caused some public concern. For example, British media have highlighted 'pioneering policy' enabling disabled teenagers to form intimate and sexual relationships at a post-16 college (Asthana, 2007), and on the other hand, we see a mother who defended her right to have her disabled 15-year-old daughter's womb removed (Bowcott, 2007). On this basis I am compelled to think about who has the rights and the mental capacity to be sexually and intimately active, to mother, and ultimately to make decisions about their own body. In addition to this, and in the context of surveillance, Carabine (2004: 147) argues that generally parents and professional carers have a great deal of control over sexual and intimate activity, for example, by restricting where young people socialise. Parents can become over-protective and find it difficult to accept young people's needs for sexual independence (Hollomotz, 2007, 2011). Furthermore, when it comes to sexual activity and sexual health, we can see that these are governed via the politics of sex education (Alldred and David, 2007) which goes beyond parental decision-making processes (although they have a part to play). A 'preoccupation has shifted and a new agenda of personalisation, linked with choice has emerged. But this is not the same as the personalisation in Personal, Social and Health Education (PSHE), but about individualisation' (Alldred and David, 2007: 13).

Intellectually disabled people might want to pursue intimate and sexual relations, but at times could need protecting from potentially harmful, potentially abusive and negative life changing incidents (McCarthy, 1999). They could inhabit care-less spaces. Therefore I recognise the importance of friendship and close relationships, and their critical place in understanding being human, as well as the systemic violence of living with a continuous blurring of boundaries when it comes to these intimacies and personal encounters. But sexuality, and the sexual reproductive body, for intellectually disabled people is an important factor also, as the socio-political sphere relating to rights, independence, interdependence, care, sex, intimate relationships and reproduction is confusing, not least when mental capacity and best interests (MCA, 2005) come into play. Intellectually disabled adults are often infantilised and sometimes considered as being like adolescents or youths. And being youthful conjures up images of virility, good looks and energy, whereas being intellectually disabled does not. Yet, Hughes, Russell and Paterson (2005: 12) found '[d]isablity is a signifier of ugliness, tragedy, asexuality, invalidity and frailty'.

Not only is imagined youthfulness pursued as something to attain, but throughout history there has been an aversion to 'difficult' bodies, especially those bodies that include intellectual impairment (or those that lack social graces). Often this aversion was, and still is, based on disgust, fear or the unknown. Significantly, underpinning some of these issues around sex and intimacy for intellectually disabled people is a deep psychic aversion to dirty, uncivilised sexual bodies (Douglas, 1966; Shakespeare, 1994) and a desire to prevent reproduction amongst inferior, or 'less that human' beings, under the political umbrella of 'protection': protection of the vulnerable, but more significantly protection of the human race (Carabine, 2004; Chadwick, 1987; Gunn, 1994; Priestley, 2003). This is deeply worrying in that it smacks of 'modern eugenics', 'weak eugenics' (Shakespeare, 1998), or 'newgenics' (Ledger et al., in press). Intellectually disabled people might not always want to have sex, or understand sex and intimate relationships; they might actually want lots of sex, or simply to have friendships. None of this is reason enough to eliminate opportunities to pursue a sexual and intimate relationship, friendship or involvement in political and citizenship discourse (Lawson, 2005; McCarthy, 1999; Shakespeare 2006).

Notably, Michel Foucault analysed crime, sex, sanity and health to ground an archaeology of what could be described as the experience of an institutionalisation of the self, based on the 'problematic' or the 'abnormal'. He claimed that during the nineteenth century there was a sanitation process, to clean up sexual and social behaviour, physical and mental health. All were categorised into 'boxes' that separated them from one another, initiated separate systems of identification and analysis, and eventually 'treated' the individual. The individual would be placed under the surveillance of appropriate 'experts' adhering to a normalisation process. According to Foucault, in the seventeenth century,

> Sexual practices had little need of secrecy [...] Codes regulating the coarse, the obscene, and the indecent were quite lax compared to those of the nineteenth century. It was a time of direct gestures, shameless discourse, and open transgressions, when anatomies were shown and intermingled at will, and knowing children hung about amid the laughter of adults: it was a period when bodies 'made a display of themselves'.
>
> (Foucault, 1990: 3)

What of sex and the sexual body today? In the twenty-first century, what is it that makes individuals and groups of people withdraw, or prohibit public displays of sexual behaviour or sexual activity? Is it against sexual 'deviance'?

Or is it about the role of normalisation? Normalisation, according to Carabine (2004), is a process defining appropriate and acceptable behaviour, operating in a regulatory capacity and producing 'differentiating effects and fragmented impacts which are in turn variously regulatory, penalizing or affirmative in respect to different groups' (Carabine, 2004: 38), all of which has an impact on intellectually disabled people and their sexual activity, relationship status, and opportunities for reproduction and childrearing.

In my previous research, a mother's description of (and aversion to) the dribbling head banging children in a 'special needs' school was graphic and emotive, as she said, 'I straight away thought, "oh my god these are physically and mentally handicapped". Excuse the expression but they were dribbling, their eyes were rolling' (Rogers, 2007a: 48). This was not a 'one off' example, but is a common theme in relating to and with other 'obviously' disabled children and the potential 'contagious' effect (although it could be argued that a child might emulate socially inappropriate behaviours, of course). It was clear in this research that the mother did not want her child (identified as having verbal dyspraxia) associating with those 'uncivilised others'. Shakespeare recognises this repulsion towards 'animality', or disability, and notes that

> the fear and loathing – that disability has for human beings is because impairment represents the physicality and animality of human existence. Nature is the enemy, women are the enemy, black people are the enemy, disabled people are the enemy.
>
> (Shakespeare, 1994: 296)

In thinking further about this repulsion, it might be considered that to be 'normal' goes beyond a project of 'normalisation', as proposed by Wolfensberger (see Race, 2003) and others, and moves onto a place in the social psyche where fear and disgust lie dormant, waiting to explode in human actions and reactions that often display aversion or even prejudice.

Discussing normalisation further, Galton named the project of human improvement eugenics, using a word he claimed was used in the Greek vocabulary to mean 'good in birth' or 'noble in heredity'. It was about removing the undesirables and 'multiplying the desirables' (Kevles, 1992: 5) and he 'advised interference in human propagation so as to increase the frequency of socially good genes in the population and decrease that of bad ones' (Kevles, 1992: 9; see also Pilnick, 2002). Of course, what really happened was that those deemed capable of 'good breeding' were encouraged to reproduce. Moreover, sterilisation was encouraged for those considered unfit to parent, and in the United States by the late 1920s 'some two dozen American states had framed such laws, often with the help of the Eugenics Record Office, and enacted them' (Kevles, 1992: 10). The control and regulation of sexual activity and procreation are apparent, both explicitly and implicitly (Carabine, 2004; Gunn, 1994; Priestley, 2003). Philosophers, sociologists and scientists continue to question what it is and what it means to be human. Scientific advances promote foetus modifications that 'enable the elimination of genes which are believed to pre-dispose people to certain illnesses. [...] Later these practices may even be extended in an attempt to improve intelligence, appearance, athleticism and behaviour' (Dickens 2001: 105). This has all had a dehumanising impact on intellectually disabled people, their families and their everyday life. Ultimately normalisation is unproductive, care-less and de-humanising as it leads to justifications on whether people live or die.

Concluding remarks

I would like to position intellectually disabled people at the centre of an agenda where their bodies, lives, and desires to have friendships, sexual relations and intimacy are critically examined within a care ethics model of disability. What I have found is that relationships and sexuality, and pleasure and intimacy, are characteristics of human life. These might change and develop through having control, or not, over a number of aspects of life, such as social and geographical mobility, dating and leisure, emotions and relationships, and reproductive life and the body. Moreover, despite work being carried out in the area, I would identify that there is some way to go setting the sexuality agenda for and with intellectually disabled people. It is also evident that in sexuality research generally there has not been enough work done when it comes to intellectual disability and relationships and the importance of friendships (intimate or otherwise), and we have not gone far enough in understanding reproductive control or pleasure. Furthermore, little research has been carried out in restricted institutional settings, and those who work with intellectually disabled people have not told their stories about sexuality and intimacy. This is currently being redressed (see Rogers, in press).

The assumed position of a relationship norm, and then how the loss of that (whether real or imagined) is played out and experienced in a caring, care-full and relational way for some researchers and family members (or carers), is evident. Importantly, intellectually disabled people do not often get what they desire, for example, love, marriage and friends. Furthermore, intellectually disabled people feel lonely and want relationships just like their non-disabled peers (Henderson et al., 2007). However, they do not necessarily have the same social, psycho-social or geographical mobility. Also, cultural scripts around relationships and intimacy are played out on the television and these images feed into how the wider public perception of intellectual disability and relationships is played out and understood. How I understand it is that intellectually disabled people are perceived as vulnerable, pitiful, tragic, angelic or heroic. In a way we can see then how this negatively impacts how intellectually disabled people might be understood when it comes to their desires and pleasures. I understand pleasure for intellectually disabled people is widely derided due to their assumed angelic or devilish nature. This is not unusual as the 'childlike' or 'predatory' intellectually disabled adult is posi-tioned as weak, vulnerable, morally fractured, lascivious and so on. As it is, there has been little care-full support for intimacy and friendship, no less procreation. This is a result of decades of stigmatisation, marginalisation and systemic violence as commonly held beliefs see intellectually disabled people as a 'parasitic, predatory class, never capable of self-support or of managing their own affairs' and they ought not 'be allowed to marry or become a parent [...] Certain families should become extinct. Parenthood is not for all' (Pfeiffer, 2006: 83). This narrative from the early twentieth century is not too dissimilar to some of the remarks levied at intellectually disabled people in the current news, from rights to earn a viable living (Withnall, 2014) to whether or not they ought to be born (Walker and Quinn, 2012). These assumptions are deeply care-less and my call for a care ethics model of disability, building through education and mothering, would benefit sexual politics in an attempt to promote a more caring and care-full society.

Notes

1 Children and adults alike on the autistic spectrum are often accused of having no emotional connection. I would suggest they just do it differently (see Shakespeare, 2006: 169).
2 Ricky Gervais, when interviewed about whether Derek has a learning disability, was incredulous, but I would argue it is clear this is a representation of intellectual disability. However, Gervais said he is just like anyone else, but kinder with a more open heart.

6   Concluding remarks

Introduction

I started this book with a quote about imagining, so imagining a society that is so bad, so care-less, so inhumane is unthinkable, and yet as we understand it, many of us live in such societies. Yet the imagining, or the 'spectacle is not a collection of images, but a social relation among people, mediated by images' (Debord, 1977: 1). This relation to images, to people, is all very real when day-to-day challenges thwart care-full moments, care-full spaces. Throughout this book I have spelled out that humans are relational beings, and as humans we have varied interpretations of images and interactions, and as such how we interact with each other, and images mediate relationships. Stuart Hall and his colleagues (2013: xvii) understand culture as embodying shared meanings, and say 'language is the privileged medium in which we "make sense" of things'. Images and representations ought to be taken seriously in researching social life, as 'the social conditions and effects of visual objects need to be considered' (Allan 2012: 78) and 'researchers need to account for their own particular ways of looking at images' (Allan 2012: 78). We understand by hearing stories told; it is not simply visual images that make meaning. Creative narratives, social media and news stories also perpetuate or repudiate cultural norms. How we interpret a painting, photograph, story, television show, or stories via social media is always based on our own imaginings. Therefore we look at and process an image, a story, an icon, before words escape, by seeing and imagining. Indeed, the way we process and interact with an image or story is reliant on our own culture, norms, individual and collective experiences (Hall, Evans and Nixon, 2013).

What some might imagine, or make meaning of, when they see an image or hear a story about an intellectually disabled person in particular circumstances, such as participating in further education, going to regular school, starring in a theatrical performance, having sex, becoming a mother/father, gaining paid employment, running a marathon, perpetrating a crime or being a victim of crime, for example, might refute or confirm a set of beliefs already held by the person interacting with that image or story told. It is at this very relational moment(s) with a story or image that the implementation of a care ethics model of disability is vital. Not least because the socio-political caring sphere is care-less, as social intolerance and aversion to difficult differences are implicitly and explicitly played out on a global stage and at a deeply psycho-social level. This plays into the hands of the emotional and practical caring spheres. The evidence of such carelessness is documented throughout this book. For example, in the extreme I identify the care-less killing field which I can situate within the socio-political sphere. I also recognise the care-less institutional spaces that populate, to an extent the emotional and practical caring spheres, although as I have highlighted they do indeed relate to each other in complex ways.

The caring spheres: a care ethics model of disability

Here I simply want to reflect upon care-less spaces that I have already identified, but with a caveat that the caring spheres do not exist in a vacuum. I merely want to ponder the question, who will care, be caring and maintain care-full practices. Below are examples:

The care-less killing fields: the socio-political caring sphere

The Care System

- LB and 'Death by Indifference' – Who is caring for those who go into care?

The Community

- Murder and Suicide – Who is caring for those in the local community? What makes someone so desperate to take the life of their child and their own?

The Media

- Denial in 'I did it all for charity': caring 'about' not 'for' and 'with' is problematic. Who is care-full in storying?

The care-less institutional space: the emotional and practical caring spheres

The Playground

- Loneliness, 'I'm the mother with the boy with ADHD' – Who is caring with the mother and the child?

The Criminal Justice System

- Following and not following the rules: 'We did everything by the book' and 'It wasn't me'. Who is care-full in legal procedure? Who will do this caring?

The School

- They call it 'inclusive education', and 'I'm just a bloody retard' –
  What does a care-full institution look like and who is a caring leader?

I have emphasised throughout that all three caring spheres interact in complex ways and that is exactly why we need a care ethics model of disability. Enforcing caring is impossible. Imposing sanctions that coerce or compel people to relate to another in a caring and care-full manner will not work. 'But societies can work to establish the conditions in which these relationships can thrive' (Lynch, Baker and Lyons, 2009: 2). More than this, though: people are human beings, all people, with all their differences and impairments. We must enable caring across all institutions, such as education, the criminal justice system, the family, as well as fundamentally transform the psycho-social responses to those who are intellectually impaired – they are not less than human. 'There is no escaping the issue of care' (Herring, 2013: 328), but if we can do this, then we can do anything.

Behind the image: the significance of the psycho-social within a care ethics model of disability

I recognise that the most difficult aspect of a care ethics model of disability is to alter the deeply embedded psycho-social responses to an intellectually disabled human being, whether that is due to lack of economic productivity, fear of impairment and mortality, or shaming and disgust. However, some stories and images that are told and retold make them part of a greater socio-political and then psycho-social narrative. Broadly, what some might imagine, or make meaning of, when they see an image of a dribbling disabled person wearing a suit, an obese person eating a burger and smoking a cigarette, a healthy looking refugee, or a Muslim woman wearing a hijab and holding hands with a white woman in Western dress can conflate, refute or confirm a set of beliefs already held by the person interacting with that image. Hall and his colleagues (2013: xvii) understand culture as being about shared meanings, and say that 'language is the privileged medium in which we "make sense" of things'. We are left to interpret these images and imaginings, to an extent. I question the notion that language is privileged, as language comes after seeing, although it does operate as a 'representational system' (Hall, Evans and Nixon, 2013: xvii) with signs and symbols, and therefore is also critical in our image processing and meaning-making, but seeing consequently impacts upon our collective interpretations. So, for example, as has been set out in the previous chapters, collective interpretations of 'choosing' not to have a disabled baby rather than what it means to live with a disabling condition, understanding messages about the 'good guys' rather than the violated young woman, or following an education pathway that is exclusionary, find their way into collective action and the social-psyche, leaving us in care-less spaces.

Collective interpretation (or action) has proved tragic in some circumstances as groups have at best been stigmatised and at worst killed and abused, sometimes en masse (see Bauman, 1989; Davis, 1995, 2006; Goodley, 2014; Nussbaum, 2004; Oliver, 1990). It is these images, whether the vehicle is fiction or news media, books or film, documentaries or soaps, social media or billboards, photographs or paintings, that have provoked and seeped into meaning-making for and about intellectually disabled people. This is largely due to the fact that the stories told and the characters portrayed are flawed, often suffering, commonly pitied, and, at best, seen as the moral compass or a joke – the comedic element or light relief. Undeniably, intellectually disabled people have been the butt of jokes for decades, indeed centuries if we include 'live drama' in the form of public displays of foolery in the middle ages to 'freak shows' in the nineteenth century (Barnes and Mercer, 2003; Garland Thomson, 1996). In more recent years, as different genres are played out, we see foolery and entertainment at the cost of intellectually disabled people. For example, the shows I have spoken about at the beginning of this book are examples of such 'entertainment'. While social justice for physically impaired people has come a long way (but there is still a way to go), intellectually disabled people are often not able to 'speak' out for themselves and are not always able to understand the meaning of their injustice (even though they feel and experience it), especially for those with profound and multiple intellectual impairments (Vorhaus, 2016). As has been acknowledged, viewing and representing disability are a part of mainstream society now. Moreover, the audience reach covers millions globally from large charity telethons and festival events (pity parties) to viewing disability via blockbusting television dramas such as *Breaking Bad* and *Game of Thrones* (Cremin, 2012; Haller, 2010). This influence is global and infects the socio-political caring sphere via the psycho-social. It is here, through the lens of the visual 'norm', the intellectual 'norm', the familial 'norm' and the sexual/relationship 'norm' that I find a raft of care-less spaces that are in need of transforming.

Nevertheless, there are some stories and images that are told and re-told, making them part of this collective interpretation and then action. So, for example, stories and images about intellectual disability and exclusion, heroism, violence, vulnerability and so on are often understood and interpreted in relation to inequality, prejudice and injustice. As highlighted in previous chapters, social networks, institutional practices, media narratives and visual images often discount, degrade, victimise and misrepresent, and can find the stigmatised, marked other, inferior, shameful, defective, monstrous and disturbing (Carrabine, 2014; Garland Thomson, 1996; Haller, 2010; Shildrick, 2002). For many individuals and communities, representations (fact/fiction, virtual, written or visual) are the only lens into particular 'realities' – so in this case, intellectually disabled people's lives and those of their families – as millions of people blog, tweet and narrate their stories, virtually or actually interact with 'friends', and individually and collectively consume and binge on blockbusting television shows/events (Carrabine, 2012; Enns and Smit, 2001; Haller, 2010;

Hevey, 1992, 2006). When it comes to disability the images portrayed and stories told are tragic, heroic, villainous and above or beneath humanity, For intellectually disabled people their story is one of horror – not like us – or not like we want to be. The irrational, erratic, slow and unintelligent (sub)human is to be feared as reason and rationality are revered.

If this care-lessness, injustice and misrepresentation is the case, can we eradicate invidious explicit and implicit forms of disablism by understanding how intellectually disabled people are embedded in the emotional, practical and socio-political spheres via a care ethics model of disability, and in understanding this, destroy discrimination, marginalisation and forms of dehumanising practices that occur, such as implicit and explicit violence and pitying gazes? As it is, according to Goffman (1990: 15), 'the person with a stigma is not quite human' and there are many who suggest that disabled people are better off dead or better still, not even born (Kittay, 2010; Riley II, 2005). Intellectually disabled people are stigmatised, but the assumed worth-lessness of life based on levels of pain, discomfort and everyday disadvantage seems to be enough to suggest that they might be better off dead. We would not say this about particular ethnic/racial groups, those living in poverty, gay people, or women – necessarily. Moreover, we do not have to search too far to find certain killing fields (Bauman, 1989) outside of intellectual disability. But it is caring, ethical and just that we critically understand the ways in which intellectually disabled people are represented and related to, and it is for all of us to organise. The care ethics model of disability set out in Chapter 2, and developed throughout the book, is just the beginning.

Bibliography

Adams, R. and Shepherd, J. (2013) 'Michael Gove proposes longer school day and shorter holidays'. Available from: http://www.theguardian.com/politics/2013/apr/18/michael-gove-longer-school-day-holidays (accessed 5 August 2015).

Adams, R. and Shepherd, J. (2014) 'Teachers spend less than half their working week in the classroom'. Available from: http://www.theguardian.com/education/2014/jun/25/teachers-classroom-working-week-england-survey (accessed 5 August 2015).

Adorno, T., Benjamin, W., Bloch, B. and Lukacs, G. (2007 [1977]) *Aesthetics and Politics*. London: Verso.

Ahmed, S. (2010) 'Secrets and silence in feminist research', in R. Ryan-Flood and R. Gill (eds) *Secrecy and Silence in the Research Process: Feminist Reflections*. Oxon: Routledge.

Allan, A. (2012) 'Doing ethnography and using visual methods', in S. Bradford and F. Cullen (eds) *Research and Research Methods for Youth Practitioners*. London: Routledge.

Allan, J. (1999a) *Actively Seeking Inclusion: Pupils with Special Educational Needs in Mainstream Schools*. London: Falmer Press.

Allan, J. (1999b) 'I don't need this: Acts of transgression by students with special educational needs', in K. Ballard (ed.) *Inclusive Education: International Voices on Disability and Justice*. London: Falmer Press, pp. 67–80.

Allan, J. (2003a) *Inclusion, Participation and Democracy: What is the Purpose?* London: Kluwer Academic Publishers.

Allan, J. (2003b) 'Daring to think otherwise? Educational policy making in the new Scottish Parliament', in J. Allan (ed.) *Inclusion, Participation and Democracy: What is the Purpose?* London: Kluwer Academic Publishers, pp. 179–194.

Allan, J. (2005) 'Inclusion as an ethical project', in S. Tremain (ed.) *Foucault and the Government of Disability*. USA: The University of Michigan Press, pp. 281–297.

Allan, J. (2010a) *Rethinking Inclusive Education: The Philosophers of Difference in Practice*. The Netherlands: Springer.

Allan, J. (2010b) 'The sociology of disability and the struggle for inclusive education', *British Journal of Sociology of Education*, 31(5): 603–620.

Alldred, P. and David, M. (2007) *Get Real About Sex: The Politics and Practice of Sex Education*. Berkshire: Open University Press.

Alur, M. (2010) 'Family perspectives: parents in partnership', in Rose, R. (ed.) *Confronting Obstacles to Inclusion: International Responses to Developing Inclusive Education*. Oxon: Routledge and Nasen, pp. 61–74.

Arendt, H. (1998 [1958]) *The Human Condition*. London: University of Chicago Press.

Asthana, A. (2007) 'Meet Tyran and Leanne – they learnt of love and sex in a school for the disabled', *guardian.co.uk*. Available from: http://www.theguardian.com/global/2007/oct/07/anushkaasthana.uknews (accessed 8 October 2015).

Banks, S. (in press) '"Knowing me, knowing you": Disability support worker as emotional mediator?' *Sexualities*.

Barnes, C. (1992) *Disabling Imagery and the Media*. Halifax: BCODP and Ryburn Publishing Limited.

Barnes, M. (2006) *Caring and Social Justice*. Basingstoke: Palgrave Macmillan.

Barnes, C. and Mercer, G. (2003) *Disability*. Cambridge: Polity Press.

Barton, L. (2006) (ed.) *Overcoming Disabling Barriers: 18 Years of Disability and Society*. London: Routledge.

Bauman, Z. (1989) *Modernity and the Holocaust*. Cambridge: Polity Press.

Bauman, Z. (2003) *Liquid Love*. Cambridge: Polity Press.

Bauman, Z. (2007) *Consuming Life*. Cambridge: Polity Press.

Bauman, Z. (2011) *Collateral Damage: Social Inequalities in a Global Age*. Cambridge: Polity Press.

Bawden, A. and Campbell, D. (2012) 'NHS accused over deaths of disabled patients', *The Guardian online*. Available from: http://www.theguardian.com/society/2012/jan/02/nhs-accused-disabled-patient-deaths (accessed 21 August 2013).

BBC News (2010) 'Woman admits killing autistic son, 12, with bleach', *bbc.co.uk*. Available from: http://www.bbc.com/news/uk-england-london-11758290 (accessed 8 October 2015).

BBC (2010) *Tormented Lives*. BBC. Rosa Monckton.

Beck, U. (1992) *Risk Society: Towards a New Modernity*. London: Sage.

Beck, U. and Beck-Gernsheim, E. (1995) *The Normal Chaos of Love*. Cambridge: Polity Press.

Beckett, A. (2006) *Citizenship and Vulnerability: Disability and Issues of Social and Political Engagement*. Houndmills: Palgrave Macmillan.

Beckett, A., Ellison, N., Barrett, S. and Shah, S. (2010) '"Away with the fairies?" Disability within primary-age children's literature', *Disability and Society*, 25(3): 373–338.

Benjamin, S. (2002) *The Micropolitics of Inclusive Education*. Buckingham: Open University Press.

Berger, J. (1972) *Ways of Seeing*. London: Penguin Books.

Berube, M. (2010) 'Equality, freedom, and/or justice for all: A response to Martha Nussbaum', in E. F. Kittay and L. Carson (eds) *Cognitive Disability and its Challenge to Moral Philosophy*. West Sussex: Wiley-Blackwell, pp. 97–110.

Block, P. (2000) 'Sexuality, fertility, and danger: Twentieth-century images of women with cognitive disabilities', *Sexuality and Disability*, 18(4): 239–254.

Bowcott, O. (2007) 'Mother defends hysterectomy for disabled daughter', *guardian.co.uk*. Available from: http://www.theguardian.com/news/2007/oct/08/medicineandhealth.uknews (accessed 8 October 2007).

Boyne, J. (2006) *The Boy in the Striped Pyjamas*. London: David Fickling Books.

Bowlby, S., McKie, L., Gregory, S. and Macpherson, I. (2010) *Interdependency and Care over the Lifecourse*. London: Routledge.

Braun, D. (2001) 'Perspectives on parenting', in P. Foley, J. Roche and S. Tucker (eds) *Children in Society: Contemporary Theory, Policy and Practice*. Basingstoke: Palgrave, pp. 239–248.

Carabine, J. (2004) (ed.) *Sexualities: Personal Lives and Social Policy*. Milton Keynes: Open University Press.

Carlile, A. (2011) 'Docile bodies or contested space? Working under the shadow of permanent exclusion', *International Journal of Inclusive Education*, 15(3): 303–316.

Carlson, L. (2005) 'Docile bodies, docile minds: Foucauldian reflections on mental retardation', in S. Tremain (ed.) *Foucault and the Government of Disability*. Michigan, USA: University of Michigan Press, pp. 133–152.

Carlson, L. (2010) *The Faces of Intellectual Disability: Philosophical Reflections*. Bloomington, USA: Indiana University Press.

Carlson, L. and Kittay, E. F. (2010) 'Introduction: Rethinking philosophical presumptions in light of cognitive disability', in E. F. Kittay and L. Carson (eds) *Cognitive Disability and its Challenge to Moral Philosophy*. West Sussex: Wiley-Blackwell, pp. 1–26.

Carrabine, E. (2012) 'Just images: Aesthetics, ethics and visual criminology', *British Journal of Criminology*, 52: 463–489.

Carrabine, E. (2014) 'Seeing things: Violence, voyeurism and the camera', *Theoretical Criminology*, 18(2): 134–158.

Cassidy, S. (2015) '"Mate crime" replacing hate crime as children with Asperger's and autism increasingly being abused and robbed by so-called friends', *The Independent*. Available from: http://www.independent.co.uk/news/uk/crime/mate-crime-replacing-hate-crime-as-children-with-aspergers-and-autism-increasingly-being-abused-and-robbed-by-socalled-friends-10383677.html (accessed 14 July 2015).

Chadwick, R. (1987) 'The perfect baby: Introduction', in R. Chadwick (ed.) *Ethics, Reproduction and Genetic Control*. London: Routledge, pp. 93–135.

Cigman, R. (2007) *Included or Excluded? The Challenge of the Mainstream for some SEN Children*. Oxon: Routledge.

Cohen, S. (2001) *States of Denial: Knowing about Atrocities and Suffering*. Cambridge: Polity Press.

Condry, R. (2007) *Families Shamed: The Consequences of Crime for Relatives of Serious Offenders*. Cullompton: Willan Publishing.

Cooper, L. and Rogers, C. (2015) 'Mothering and "insider" dilemmas: Feminist sociologists in the research process', *Sociological Research Online*, 20(2): 5.

Coward, R. (1997) 'The heaven and hell of mothering: Mothering and ambivalence in the mass media', in W. Hollway and B. Featherstone (eds) *Mothering and Ambivalence*. London: Routledge, pp. 111–118.

Craft, A. (1994) *Sexuality and Learning Disabilities*. London: Routledge.

Craib, I. (1994) *The Importance of Disappointment*. London: Routledge.

Cremin, C. (2012) 'The social logic of late capitalism: Guilt fetishism and the culture of crisis industry', *Cultural Sociology*, 6(1): 45–60.

Crozier, G. and Reay, D. (2004) (eds) *Activating PARTICIPATION: Parents and Teachers Working Towards Partnership*. Stoke on Trent: Trentham Books.

Culpitt, I. (1999) *Social Policy and Risk*. London: Sage Publications.

Darke, A. (2004) 'The changing face of representations of disability in the media', in J. Swain, S. French, C. Barnes and C. Thomas (eds) *Disabling Barriers – Enabling Environments*. London: Sage Publications.

Davis, L. J. (1995) *Enforcing Normalcy: Disability, Deafness, and the Body*. London: Verso.

Davis, L. J. (2006) 'The end of identity politics and the beginning of dismodernism: On disability as an unstable category', in L. J. Davis (ed.) *The Disability Studies Reader*. London: Routledge.

Davis, L. J. (2006) 'Constructing normalcy: The bell curve, the novel, and the invention of the disabled body in the nineteenth century', in L. J. Davis (ed.) *The Disability Studies Reader* (2nd edn). Oxon: Routledge.

Davis, L. J. (2013) *The End of Normal: Identity in a Bicultural Era*. Michigan, USA: University of Michigan Press.

DCFS (2009) *Lamb Inquiry: Special Educational Needs and Parental Confidence*. Nottingham: Department for Children, Schools and Families.

Dean, H. (2010) *Understanding Human Need*. Bristol: The Policy Press.

Debord, G. (1977) *Society of the Spectacle*. California: AK Press.

Deng, M. (2010) 'Developing inclusive approaches to teaching and learning', in R. Rose (ed.) *Confronting Obstacles to Inclusion: International Responses to Developing Inclusive Education*. Oxon: Routledge and Nasen.

De Guimps, R. (2004) *Pestalozzi: His Life and Work*. New York: Elibron Classics.

DES (1978) 'Special Educational Needs', in *The Warnock Report*. London: Department of Education and Science.

Desjardins, M. (2012) 'The sexualized body of the child: Parents and the politics of "voluntary" sterilization of people labelled intellectually disabled', in R. McRuer and A. Mollow (eds) *Sex and Disability*. London: Duke University Press.

DfE (2010) *Every Disabled Child Matters: Spending Review 2010*. London: Department for Education.

DfEE (1996) *Education Act*. London: Department for Education and Employment.

DfES (2001a) *Code of Practice on the Identification and Assessment of Special Educational Needs*. London: Department for Education and Skills.

DfES (2001b) *Special Educational Needs and Disability Act*. London: Department for Education and Skills.

DfES (2005) *Higher Standards, Better Schools for All: More Choice for Parents and Pupils*. London: Department of State for Education and Skills.

DfES (2007) *Every Parent Matters*. London: Department for Education and Skills.

Dickens, P. (2001) 'Linking the social and natural sciences: Is capital modifying human biology in its own image?' *Sociology*, 35(1): 93–110.

Didi-Huberman, G. (2003) *Invention of Hysteria: Charcot and the Photographic Iconography of the Salpêtrière*. London: MIT Press.

Doddington, K., Jones, R. S. P. and Miller, B. Y. (1994) 'Are attitudes to people with learning disabilities negatively influenced by charity advertising?' *Disability and Society*, 9(2): 207–222.

Donzelot, J. (1979) *The Policing of Families*. London: John Hopkins University Press.

Doucet, A. (2006) *Do Men Mother?* Toronto: University of Toronto Press.

Doucet, A. and Mauthner, N. (2013) 'Tea and tupperware: Mommy blogging as care, work, and consumption', in C. Rogers and S. Weller (eds) *Critical Approaches to Care: Understanding Caring Relations, Identities and Cultures*. London: Routledge.

Douglas, M. (1966) *Purity and Danger*. London: Routledge.

Douglas, S. J. and Michaels, M. W. (2005) *The Mommy Myth: The Idealisation of Motherhood and how it has Undermined all Women*. New York: Free Press.

Duncan, S. and Edwards, R. (1999) *Lone Mothers, Paid Work and Gendered Moral Rationalities*. London: Macmillan.

Earle, S., Bartholomew, C. and Komaromy, C. (eds) (2009) *Making Sense of Death and Dying and Bereavement: An Anthology*. London: Sage and Open University Press.

Earle, S. and Letherby, G. (2007) 'Conceiving time? Women who do or do not conceive', *Sociology of Health and Illness*, 29(2): 233–250.

ECM (2004) *Every Child Matters: Change for Children*. Nottingham: Department for Education and Skills.

Enns, A. and Smit, C. (2001) *Screening Disability*. Oxford: University Press of America.

Feely, M. (in press) 'Sexual surveillance and control in a community based intellectual disability service', *Sexualities*.

Finkelstein, V. (1996) 'Outside, "Inside Out"', *Coalition*, April, 30–36.

Fish, R. (in press) '"They've said I'm vulnerable with men": Doing sexuality on locked wards', *Sexualities*.

Florian, L. and Rouse, M. (2010) 'Teachers' professional learning and inclusive practice', in R. Rose (ed.) *Confronting Obstacles to Inclusion: International Responses to Developing Inclusive Education*. Oxon: Routledge and Nasen.

Forna, A. (1998) *Mother of all Myths: How Society Moulds and Constrains Mothers*. London: Harper Collins Publishers.

Foucault, M. (1984) 'On the genealogy of ethics: An overview of work in progress', in P. Rabinow (ed.) *The Foucault Reader*. New York: Pantheon.

Foucault, M. (1989) *Madness and Civilisation: A History of Insanity in the Age of Reason*. London: Routledge.

Foucault, M. (1990) *The History of Sexuality, Volume 1: An Introduction*. London: Penguin.

Foucault, M. (1991) *Discipline and Punish: The Birth of the Prison*. London: Penguin.

Foucault, M. (2003) *The Birth of the Clinic*. London: Routledge.

Foucault, M. and Faubion, J. (2002) *Power: The Essential Works of Michel Foucault 1954–1984*. London: Penguin.

Frank, A. W. (1995) *The Wounded Storyteller: Body, Illness and Ethics*. London: University of Chicago Press.

Frank, A. W. (2001) 'Can we research suffering?' *Qualitative Health Research*, 11(3): 353–362.

Frost, J., Bradley, H., Levitas, R., Smith, L. and Garcia, J. (2007) 'The loss of possibility: Scientisation of death and the special case of early miscarriage', *Sociology of Health and Illness*, 29(7): 1003–1022.

Friedman, M. (1995) 'Beyond caring: The de-moralization of gender', in V. Held (ed.) *Justice and Care: Essential Readings in Feminist Ethics*. Colorado, USA: Westview Press.

Frierson, P. R. (2013) *What is the Human Being?* London: Routledge.

Furedi, F. (2006) *Culture of Fear: Revisited*. London: Continuum.

Gabb, J. (2008) *Researching Intimacy in Families*. Houndmills: Palgrave Macmillan.

Garland Thomson, R. (ed.) (1996) *Freakery: Cultural Spectacles of the Extraordinary Body*. London: New York University Press.

Gartner, A. and Joe, T. (eds) (1987) *Images of the Disabled, Disabling Images*. New York: Praeger Publishers.

Geertz, C. (1973) *The Interpretation of Cultures*. New York: Basic Books.

Gibran, K. (1996 [1923]) *The Prophet*. Hertfordshire: Wordsworth Editions.

Gillespie-Sells, K., Hill, M. and Robbins, B. (1998) *She Dances to Different Drums: Research into Disabled Women's Sexuality*. London: Kings Fund Publishing.

Gillies, V. (2007) *Marginalised Mothers: Exploring Working-class Experiences of Parenting*. London: Routledge.

Gillies, V. (2012) '"Inclusion" through exclusion: A critical account of new behaviour management practices in schools', in Y. Taylor (ed.) *Educational Diversity: The Subject of Difference and Different Subjects*. Houndmills: Palgrave Macmillan.

Gillies, V. (forthcoming) *Pushed to the Edge: Inclusion and Behaviour Support in Schools*. Bristol: Policy Press.

Gillies, V. and Robinson, Y. (2010) 'Managing emotions in research with challenging pupils', *Ethnography and Education*, 5(1): 97–110.

Gillies, V. and Robinson, Y. (2013) 'At risk pupils and the "caring" curriculum', in C. Rogers and S. Weller (eds) *Critical Approaches to Care: Understanding Caring Relations, Identities and Cultures*. London: Routledge.

Gilligan, C. (1993 [1982]) *In a Different Voice: Psychological Theory and Women's Development*. Cambridge, USA: Harvard University Press.

Goffman, E. (1990 [1963]) *Stigma: Notes on the Management of Spoiled Identity*. London: Penguin.

Goldring, M. (2012) 'The NHS must accelerate its reforms on treating learning disabled patients', *The Guardian online*. Available from: http://www.theguardian.com/society/2012/feb/15/change-nhs-learning-disabled-patients-accelerate (accessed 21 August 2013).

Goodley, D. (2014) *Dis/ability Studies: Theorizing Disablism and Ableism*. Oxon: Routledge.

Graham, H. (1983) 'Caring: a labour of love', in J. Finch and D. Groves (eds) *A Labour of Love*. London: Routledge & Kegan Paul.

Gunn, M. (1994) 'Competency and consent: The importance of decision-making', in A. Craft (ed.) *Sexuality and Learning Disabilities*. London: Routledge, pp. 116–134.

Habermas, J. (2003) *The Future of Human Nature*. Cambridge: Polity Press.

Hall, S. (2013) 'The work of representation', in S. Hall, J. Evans and S. Nixon (eds) *Representation*. London: Sage Publications.

Hall, S., Evans, J. and Nixon, S. (eds) (2013) *Representation*. London: Sage Publications.

Haller, B. (2010) *Representing Disability in an Ableist World*. Louisville: Advocado Press.

Haller, B., Ralph, S. and Zaks, Z. (2010) 'Confronting obstacles to inclusion: How the US news media report disability', in R. Rose (ed.) *Confronting Obstacles to Inclusion: International Responses to Developing Inclusive Education*. Oxon: Routledge and Nasen, pp. 9–30.

Hartley, C. (2009) 'An inclusive contractualism: Obligations to the mentally disabled', in K. Brownlee and A. Cureton (eds) *Disability and Disadvantage*. New York: Oxford University Press, pp. 138–161.

Held, V. (ed.) (1995) *Justice and Care: Essential Readings in Feminist Ethics*. Oxford: Westview Press.

Held, V. (2006) *The Ethics of Care: Personal, Political and Global*. Oxford: Oxford University Press.

Henderson, S., Holland, J., McGrellis, S., Sharpe, S. and Thomson, R. (2007) *Inventing Adulthoods: A Biographical Approach to Youth Transitions*. London: Sage Publications.

Herring, J. (2013) *Caring and the Law*. Oxford: Hart Publishing Ltd.

Hevey, D. (1992) *The Creatures Time Forgot: Photography and Disability Imagery*. London: Routledge.

Hevey, D. (2006) 'The enfreakment of photography', in L. J. Davis (ed.) *The Disability Studies Reader* (2nd edn). Oxon: Routledge.

Hillyer, B. (1993) *Feminism and Disability*. London: University of Oklahoma Press.

Hochschild, A. (1983) *The Managed Heart: Commercialization of Human Feeling*. California, USA: University of California Press.

Hodge, N. and Runswick-Cole, K. (2008) 'Problematising parent-professional partnerships in education', *Disability and Society*, 23(6): 637–647.

Hollomotz, A. (2007) 'Beyond "vulnerability": An ecological model approach to conceptualising risk of sexual violence against people with learning difficulties', *British Journal of Social Work*, 14 September.

Hollomotz, A. (2011) *Learning Difficulties and Sexual Vulnerability: A Social Approach*. London: Jessica Kingsley Publishers.

Hollway, W. (2006) *The Capacity to Care: Gender and Ethical Subjectivity*. Hove: Routledge.

Hollway, W. and Featherstone, B. (eds) (1997) *Mothering and Ambivalence*. London: Routledge.

Hooyman, N. and Gonyea, J. (1999) 'A feminist model of family care: practice and policy directions', *Journal of Women and Ageing*, 11(2/3): 149–169.

Hornby, G. (2010) 'Supporting parents and families in the development of inclusive practice', in R. Rose (ed.) *Confronting Obstacles to Inclusion: International Responses to Developing Inclusive Education*. Oxon: Routledge and Nasen, pp. 75–80.

Hornby, M. (2008) 'Mother jailed for murder of disabled daughter', 23 September, *The Independent*.

Hughes, B. (2005) 'What can a Foucauldian analysis contribute to disability theory?', in S. Tremain (ed.) *Foucault and the Government of Disability*. Michigan, USA: University of Michigan Press, pp. 78–92.

Hughes, B., McKie, L., Hopkins, D. and Watson, N. (2005) 'Love's labour's lost? Feminism, the Disabled People's Movement and an ethic of care', *Sociology*, 39(2): 259–275.

Hughes, B., Russell, R. and Paterson, K. (2005) 'Nothing to be had "off the peg": Consumption, identity and the immobilization of young disabled people', *Disability and Society*, 20(1): 3–17.

Hull, R. (2009) 'Disability and freedom', in K. Kristiansen, S. Vehmas and T. Shakespeare (eds) *Arguing about Disability: Philosophical Perspectives*. Oxon: Routledge.

Hull, R. (2009) 'Projected disability and parental responsibilities', in K. Brownlee and A. Cureton (eds) *Disability and Disadvantage*. New York: Oxford University Press, pp. 369–384.

Jackson, S. and Scott, S. (2006) 'Childhood', in G. Payne (ed.) *Social Divisions* (2nd edn). Basingstoke: Palgrave Macmillan.

James, A. and Prout, A. (1997) *Constructing and Reconstructing Childhood*. London: Routledge Falmer.

Jones, A. (2010) (ed.) *The Feminism and Visual Culture Reader* (2nd edn). Oxon: Routledge.

Jones, P. and Gillies, A. (2010) 'Engaging young children in research about an inclusion project', in R. Rose (ed.) *Confronting Obstacles to Inclusion: International Responses to Developing Inclusive Education*. Oxon: Routledge and Nasen, pp. 123–136.

Justice for LB (2015a) Available from: https://107daysofaction.wordpress.com/ (accessed 5 August 2015).

Justice for LB (2015b) Available from: https://107daysofaction.wordpress.com/2015/07/04/week-15-the-tale-of-laughing-boy-107days/ (accessed 5 August 2015).

Kehily, M. J. (2002) *Sexuality, Gender and Schooling: Shifting Agendas in Social Learning*. London: Routledge Falmer.

Kelly, L. (1988) *Surviving Sexual Violence*. Cambridge: Polity Press.

Kelly, G., Crowley, H. and Hamilton, C. (2009) 'Rights, sexuality and relationships in Ireland: "It'd be nice to be kind of trusted"', *British Journal of Learning Disabilities*, 37: 308–315.

Kevles, D. (1992) 'Out of eugenics: The historical politics of the human genome', in J. Kevles and L. Hood (eds) *The Code of Codes*. London: Harvard University Press, pp. 3–36.

Kijak, R. (2013) 'The sexuality of adults with intellectual disability in Poland', *Sexuality and Disability*, 31: 109–123.

Kempe, A. (2013) *Drama, Disability and Education*. London: Routledge.

Kim, E. (2011) 'Asexuality in disability narratives', *Sexualities*, 14(4): 479–493.

Kittay, E. F. (1999) *Love's Labor: Essays on Women, Equality, and Dependency*. New York: Routledge.

Kittay, E. F. (2005) 'Dependency, difference and the global ethic of care', *Journal of Political Philosophy*, 13(4): 443–469.

Kittay, E. F. (2010) 'The personal is philosophical is political: a philosopher and mother of a cognitively disabled person sends notes from the battlefield', in E. F. Kittay and L. Carlson (eds) *Cognitive Disability and its Challenge to Moral Philosophy*. Chichester: Wiley-Blackwell.

Kittay, E. F. and Carlson, L. (eds) (2010) *Cognitive Disability and its Challenge to Moral Philosophy*. Chichester: Wiley-Blackwell.

Kittay, E. F. with Jennings, B. and Wasunna, A. (2005) 'Dependency, difference and the global ethic of longterm care', *The Journal of Political Philosophy*, 13(4): 443–469.

Korsgaard, C. (1996) (ed.) *The Sources of Normativity*. Cambridge: Cambridge University Press.

Korsgaard, C. (2009) *Self-constitution: Agency, Identity and Integrity*. Oxford: Oxford University Press.

Kuppers, P. (2002) 'Image politics without the real: Simulacra, dandyism and disability fashion', in M. Corker and T. Shakespeare (eds) *Disability/Postmodernity: Embodying Disability Theory*. London: Continuum.

Landsman, G. H. (2009) *Reconstructing Motherhood and Disability in the Age of 'Perfect' Babies*. London: Routledge.

Lasch, C. (1991) *The Culture of Narcissism: American Life in an Age of Diminishing Expectations*. London: W. W. Norton & Company Ltd.

Lawson, W. (2005) *Sex, Sexuality and the Autistic Spectrum*. London: Jessica Kingsley Publishers Ltd.

Lawson, H. (2010) 'Beyond tokenism? Participation and "voice" for pupils with significant learning difficulites', in R. Rose (ed.) *Confronting Obstacles to Inclusion: International Responses to Developing Inclusive Education*. Oxon: Routledge and Nasen, pp. 137–151.

Ledger, S., Earle, S., Tilley, L. and Walmsley, J. (in press) 'Contraceptive decision-making and women with learning disabilities', *Sexualities*.

Lefkowitz, B. (1998) *Our Guys*. New York: First Vintage Books.

Letherby, G. (1999) 'Other than mother and mothers as others: The experience of motherhood and non-motherhood in relation to "infertility" and "involuntary childlessness"', *Women's Studies International Forum*, 22(3): 359–372.

Letherby, G. (2002) 'Childless and bereft? Stereotypes and realities in relation to "voluntary" and "involuntary" childlessness and womanhood', *Sociological Inquiry*, 72(1): 7–20.

Letherby, G. (2009) 'Experiences of miscarriage', in S. Earle, C. Bartholomew and C. Komaromy (eds) *Making Sense of Death and Dying and Bereavement: An Anthology*. London: Sage and Open University Press.

Letherby, G. and Williams, C. (1999) 'Non-motherhood: Ambivalent identities, *Feminist Studies*, 25(3): 719–728.

Levitas, R. (2001) 'Against work: A utopian incursion into social policy', *Critical Social Policy*, 21(4): 449–465.

Lewis, J. and Knijn, T. (2002) 'The politics of sex education policy in England and Wales and The Netherlands since the 1980s', *Journal of Social Policy*, 31(4): 669–694.

Longmore, P. K. (1987) 'Screening stereotypes: Images of disabled people in television and motion pictures', in A. Gartner and T. Joe (eds) *Images of the Disabled, Disabling Images*. New York: Praeger.

Luff, P. (2013) 'Reclaiming care in early childhood education and care', in C. Rogers and S. Weller (eds) *Critical Approaches to Care: Understanding Caring Relations, Identities and Cultures*. London: Routledge, pp. 18–29.

Lynch, K. (2007) 'Love labour as a distinct and non-commodifiable form of care labour', *The Sociological Review*, 55(3): 550–570.

Lynch, K., Baker, J. and Lyons, M. (eds) (2009) *Affective Equality: Love, Care and Injustice*. Houndsmill: Palgrave Macmillan.

Mahon, R. and Robinson, F. (eds) (2011) *Feminist Ethics and Social Policy: Towards a New Global Political Economy of Care*. Canada: University of British Columbia Press.

Marx, K. (2007 [1844]) *Economic and Philosophic Manuscripts of 1844*. New York: Dover Publications.

Mayall, B. (2002) *Towards a Sociology for Childhood*. Buckingham: Open University Press.

MCA (2005) *Mental Capacity Act 2005*. London: HMSO.

McCarthy, M. (1999) *Sexuality and Women with Learning Disabilities*. London: Jessica Kingsley Publishers.

McCarthy, M. (2009) '"I have the jab so I can't be blamed for getting pregnant": Contraception and women with learning disabilities', *Women's Studies International Forum*, 32: 198–208.

McCarthy, M. (2010) 'Exercising choice and control – women with learning disabilities and contraception', *British Journal of Learning Disabilities*, 38: 293–302.

McLaughlin, J., Goodley, D., Clavering, E. and Fisher, P. (2008) *Families Raising Disabled Children: Enabling Care and Social Justice*. Basingstoke: Palgrave Macmillan.

McLellan, D. (2000) *Karl Marx: Selected Writings* (2nd edn). New York: Oxford University Press.

McRuer, R. and Mollow, A. (eds) (2012) *Sex and Disability*. London: Duke University Press.

Mencap (2007) *Death by Indifference*. London: Mencap.

Mencap (2012) *Death by Indifference: 74 Deaths and Counting: A Progress Report 5 Years On*. London: Mencap.

Miller, T. (2005) *Making Sense of Motherhood: A Narrative Approach*. Cambridge: Cambridge University Press.

Miller, W. I. (1997) *The Anatomy of Disgust*. London: Harvard University Press.

Minow, M. (1991) *Making all the Difference: Inclusion, Exclusion and American Law*. New York: Cornell University Press.

de Montaigne, M. (1991 [1580]) *On Friendship*. London: Penguin.

Moore, H. L. (1996) 'Mothering and social responsibilities in a cross-cultural perspective', in E. Bortolaia Silva (ed.) *Good Enough Mothering: Feminist Perspectives on Lone Motherhood*. London: Routledge, pp. 58–75.

Morris, J. (1996) *Encounters with Strangers: Feminism and Disability*. London: The Women's Press Ltd.

Moulder, C. (2001) *Miscarriage: Women's Experiences and Needs*. London: Routledge.

Murray, P. (2000) 'Disabled children, parents and professionals: Partnership on whose Terms?' *Disability and Society*, 15(4): 683–698.

Mumsnet (2013) Available from: http://www.mumsnet.com/Talk/special_educational_needs (accessed 5 August 2015).

Mydaftlife (2013) Available from: https://mydaftlife.wordpress.com/author/sarasiobhan/ (accessed 5 August 2015).

Noddings, N. (2003 [1984]) *Caring: A Feminine Approach to Ethics and Moral Education*. London: University of California Press.

Noddings, N. (1995) 'Caring', in V. Held (ed.) *Justice and Care: Essential Readings in Feminist Ethics*. Colorado, USA: Westview Press.

Norwich, B. (2008) *Dilemmas of Difference, Inclusion and Disability*. Oxon: Routledge.

Nussbaum, M. C. (2000) *Women and Human Development*. New York: Cambridge University Press.

Nussbaum, M. C. (2004) *Hiding from Humanity: Disgust, Shame and the Law*. Oxford: Princetown University Press.

Nussbaum, M. C. (2006) *Frontiers of Justice: Disability, Nationality, Species Membership*. Connecticut, USA: First Harvard University Press.

Nussbaum, M. C. (2009) 'Education for profit, education for freedom', *Liberal Education*, Summer, 6–13.

Nussbaum, M. C. (2011) *Creating Capabilities: The Human Development Approach*. Connecticut, USA: Harvard University Press.

Nutt, L. (2013) 'Foster care in ambiguous contexts: Competing understandings of care', in C. Rogers and S. Weller (eds) *Critical Approaches to Care: Understanding Caring Relations, Identities and Cultures*. London: Routledge, pp. 122–131.

Oakley, A. (1981) 'Interviewing women', in H. Roberts (ed.) *Doing Feminist Research*. London: Routledge & Kegan Paul Ltd.

Oakley, A. (1992) *Social Support and Motherhood*. Oxford: Blackwell Publishers.

Oakley, A., McPherson, A. and Roberts, H. (1990) *Miscarriage*. London: Penguin Books.

Oliver, M. (1990) *The Politics of Disablement*. Houndmills: Palgrave Macmillan.

Oliver, M. (1996) *Understanding Disability: From Theory to Practice*. Houndmills: Palgrave.

Oliver, M. and Barnes, C. (2010) 'Disability studies, disabled people and the struggle for inclusion', *British Journal of Sociology of Education*, 31(5): 547–560.

Oliver, M. and Barnes, C. (2012) *The New Politics of Disablement*. Houndmills: Palgrave Macmillan.

O'Neill, O. (1996) 'Introduction', in C. Korsgaard (ed.) *The Sources of Normativity*. Cambridge: Cambridge University Press, pp. xi–xv

Ong-Dean, C. (2009) *Distinguishing Disability: Parents, Privilege, and Special Education*. London: University of Chicago Press.

Pahl, R. (2000) *On Friendship*. Cambridge: Polity Press.

Parker, R. (1997) 'The production and purposes of maternal ambivalence', in W. Hollway and B. Featherstone (eds) *Mothering and Ambivalence*. London: Routledge, pp. 17–36.

Pfeiffer, D. (2006) 'Eugenics and disability discrimination', in L. Barton (ed.) *Overcoming Disabling Barriers: 18 Years of Disability and Society*. London: Routledge.

Philip, G., Rogers, C. and Weller, S. (2013) 'Introduction', in C. Rogers and S. Weller (eds) *Critical Approaches to Care: Understanding Caring Relations, Identities and Cultures*. London: Routledge.

Phillips, A. (2001) 'Feminism and liberalism revisited: Has Martha Nussbaum got it right?' *Constellations*, 8(2): 249–265.

Pilnick, A. (2002) *Genetics and Society: An Introduction*. Buckingham: Open University Press.

Plummer, K. (1994) *Telling Sexual Stories: Power, Change and Social Worlds*. London: Routledge.

Plummer, K. (2001) *Documents of Life 2: An Invitation to a Critical Humanism*. London: Sage.

Plummer, K. (2003) *Intimate Citizenship: Private Decisions and Public Dialogues*. Washington, USA: University of Washington Press.

Plummer, K. (2015) *Cosmopolitan Sexualities: Hope and the Humanist Imagination*. Cambridge: Polity Press.

Priestley, M. (2003) *Disability: A Life Course Approach*. Cambridge: Polity Press.

Rabinow, P. (ed.) (1984) *The Foucault Reader*. Harmondsworth: Penguin Books.

Race, D. (2003) (ed.) *Leadership and Change in Human Services: Selected Readings from Wolf Wolfensberger*. London: Routledge.

Ramesh, R. (2011) 'UK children stuck in the "materialistic trap"', *The Guardian online*. Available from: http://www.guardian.co.uk/society/2011/sep/14/uk-children-stuck-materialistic-trap (accessed 5 August 2015).

Read, J. (2000) *Disability, the Family and Society: Listening to Mothers*. Buckingham: Open University Press.

Ribbens McCarthy, J. (2013) 'Caring after death: Issues of embodiment and relationality', in C. Rogers and S. Weller (eds) *Critical Approaches to Care: Understanding Caring Relations, Identities and Cultures*. London: Routledge, pp. 183–194.

Ribbens McCarthy, J., Edwards, R. and Gillies, V. (2003) *Making Families, Moral Tales of Parenting and Step Parenting*. Durham: Sociology Press.

Richards, D., Watson, S. L., Monger, S. and Rogers, C. (2012) 'The right to sexuality and relationships', in F. Owen, D. Griffiths and S. Watson (eds) *The Human Rights Agenda for Persons with Intellectual Disabilities*. New York: NADD Press.

Ricoeur, P. (1989) *Ricoeur: The Conflict of Interpretations*. London: Continuum Press.

Ricoeur, P. (1995) *Figuring the Sacred: Religion, Narrative and Imagination*. Minneapolis, USA: Fortress Press.

Riley II, C. (2005) *Disability and the Media: Prescriptions for Change*. Pennsylvania, USA: University Press of New England.

Robinson, F. (2011a) *The Ethics of Care: A Feminist Approach to Human Security*. Philadelphia: Temple University Press.

Robinson, F. (2011b) 'Care ethics and the transnationalization of care: Reflections on autonomy, hegemonic masculinities, and globalisation', in R. Mahon and F. Robinson (eds) *Feminist Ethics and Social Policy: Towards a New Global Political Economy of Care*. Canada: University of British Columbia Press.

Robinson, K. (2013) 'To encourage creativity, Mr Gove, you must first understand what it is'. Available from: http://www.theguardian.com/commentisfree/2013/may/17/to-encourage-creativity-mr-gove-understand (accessed 5 August 2015).

Rogers, C. (2003) 'The mother/researcher in blurred boundaries of a reflexive research process', *Auto/Biography*, XI (1&2): 47–54.

Rogers, C. (2005) *A Sociology of Parenting Children Identified with Special Educational Needs: The Private and Public Spaces Parents inhabit*. University of Essex. Unpublished PhD.

Rogers, C. (2007a) *Parenting and Inclusive Education: Discovering Difference, Experiencing Difficulty*. Houndmills: Palgrave Macmillan.

Rogers, C. (2007b) '"Disabling" a family? Emotional dilemmas experienced in becoming a parent of a learning disabled child', *British Journal of Special Education*, 34(3) 136–143.

Rogers, C. (2009a) '(S)excerpts from a life told: Sex, gender and learning disability', *Sexualities*, 12(3): 270–288.

Rogers, C. (2009b) 'Hope as a mechanism in emotional survival: Documenting miscarriage', *Auto/Biography Year Book 2009*. Nottingham: Russell Press.

Rogers, C. (2010) 'But it's not all about the sex: Mothering, normalisation and young learning disabled people', *Disability and Society*, 25(1): 63–74.

Rogers, C. (2011) 'Mothering and intellectual disability: Partnership rhetoric?' *British Journal of Sociology of Education*, 32(4): 563–581.

Rogers, C. (2013a) 'Intellectual disability and mothering: An engagement with ethics of care and emotional work', in C. Rogers and S. Weller (eds) *Critical Approaches to Care: Understanding Caring Relations, Identities and Cultures*. London: Routledge.

Rogers, C. (2013b) 'Inclusion, education and intellectual disability: A sociological engagement with Martha Nussbaum', *International Journal of Inclusive Education*, 17(9): 988–1002.

Rogers, C. (2013c) 'Mothering for life? Fractured maternal narratives, care and intellectual disability', in M. Bouvard (ed.) *Mother's of Adult Children*. New York: Lexington Press.

Rogers, C. (2014) 'Here we go…vulnerability, injustice and the criminal justice system'. Available from: https://chrissiealison.wordpress.com/2014/03/25/here-we-go-vulnerability-injustice-and-the-criminal-justice-system/ (accessed 5 August 2015).

Rogers, C. (2015) *Just Life*. Available from: https://chrissiealison.wordpress.com/ (accessed 5 August 2015).

Rogers, C. (in press) 'Intellectual disability and sexuality: On the agenda?', *Sexualities* (special issue).

Rogers, C. and Ludhra, G. (2012) 'Research ethics: Participation, social difference and informed consent', in S. Bradford and F. Cullen (eds) *Research and Research Methods for Youth Practitioners*. London: Routledge, pp. 43–63.

Rogers, C. with Tuckwell, S. (in press) 'Co-constructed research and intellectual disability: An exploration of friendship, intimacy and being human', *Sexualities*.

Rose, N. (1989) *Governing the Soul: The Shaping of the Private Self*. London: Free Association Books.

Rose, G. (2012) *Visual Methodologies*. London: Sage.

Rose, R. (ed.) (2010) *Confronting Obstacles to Inclusion: International Responses to Developing Inclusive Education*. Oxon: Routledge and Nasen.

Rose, J. and Jones, C. (1994) 'Working with parents', in A. Craft (ed.) *Sexuality and Learning Disabilities*. London: Routledge, pp. 23–49.

Roseneil, S. (2004) 'Why we should care about friends: An argument for queering the care imaginary in Social Policy', *Social Policy and Society*, 4(3): 409–419.

Ruddick, S. (1989) *Maternal Thinking: Toward a Politics of Peace*. Boston, MA: Beacon Press.

Runswick-Cole, K. (2007) '"The tribunal was the most stressful thing: more stressful than my son's diagnosis or behaviour": The experiences of families who go to the Special Educational Needs and Disability Tribunal (SENDisT)', *Disability and Society*, 22(3): 315–328.

Russell, P. (1997) 'Parents as partners: Some early impressions of the impact of the Code of Practice', in S. Wolfendale (ed.) *Working With Parents of SEN Children after the Code of Practice*. London: David Fulton Publishers, pp. 69–81.

Ryan, S. (2013a) 'About'. Available from https://mydaftlife.wordpress.com/about/ (accessed 20 July 2014).

Ryan, S. (2013b) 'The day after'. Available from: https://mydaftlife.wordpress.com/2013/07/05/ (accessed 20 July 2014).

Ryan, S. (2013c) 'Care'. Available from: https://mydaftlife.wordpress.com/2013/07/19/ (accessed 20 July 2014).

Ryan, S. (2015) 'Week 15: The tale of laughing boy #107days'. Available from: https://107daysofaction.wordpress.com/2015/07/04/week-15-the-tale-of-laughing-boy-107days/ (accessed 5 July 2015).

Ryan, S. and Runswick-Cole, K. (2008) 'Repositioning mothers: Mothers, disabled children and disability studies', *Disability and Society*, 23(3): 199–210.

Ryan, S. and Runswick-Cole, K. (2009) 'From advocate to activist? Mapping the experiences of mothers of children on the autism spectrum', *Journal of Applied Research in Intellectual Disabilities*, 22: 43–53.

Sakellariou, D. (2012) 'Sexuality and disability: A discussion on care of the self', *Sexuality and Disability*, 30: 187–197.

Sandell, R., Dodd, J. and Garland-Thomson, R. (2010) (eds) *Representing Disability: Activism and Agency in the Museum*. Oxon: Routledge.

Scheper-Hughes, N. (1992) *Death without Weeping: The Violence of Everyday Life in Brazil*. London: University of California Press.

Schwartz, D., Blue, E., McDonald, M., Giuliani, G., Weber, G., Seirup, H., Rose, S., Elkis-Albuhoff, D., Rosenfeld, J. and Perkins, A. (2010) 'Dispelling stereotypes: Promoting disability equality through film', *Disability and Society*, 25(7): 841–848.

Schwartz, K., Lutfiyya, Z. M. and Hansen, N. (2013) 'Dopey's legacy: Stereotypical portrayals of intellectual disability in the classic animated films', in J. Cheu (ed.) *Diversity in Disney Films*. North Carolina: McFarland & Company Inc. Publishers.

Sen, A. (1992) *Inequality Reexamined*. New York: Russel Sage.

Sen, A. (1999) *Development as Freedom*. New York: Knopf.

Sen, A. (2009) *The Idea of Justice*. London: Penguin.

Sevenhuijsen, S. (1998) *Citizenship and the Ethics of Care: Feminist Considerations on Justice, Morality and Politics*. London: Routledge.

Sevenhuijsen, S. (2000) 'Caring in the third way: The relation between obligation, responsibility and care in Third Way discourse', *Critical Social Policy*, 20(1): 5–37.

Sevenhuijsen, S. (2002) 'A third way? Moralities, ethics and families. An approach through the ethics of care', in A. Carling, S. Duncan and R. Edwards (eds) *Analysing Families: Morality and Rationality in Policy and Practice*. London: Routledge.

Sevenhuijsen, S. (2003) 'The place of care: The relevance of the Feminist Ethic of Care for Social Policy', *Feminist Theory*, 4(2): 179–197.

Shain, F. (2011) *The New Folk Devils: Muslim Boys and Education in England*. Stoke on Trent: Trentham Books.

Shakespeare, T. (1994) 'Cultural representation of disabled people: Dustbins for disavowal?' *Disability and Society*, 9(3): 283–299.

Shakespeare, T. (1998) 'Choices and rights: Eugenics, genetics and disability', *Disability and Society*, 13(5): 137–145.

Shakespeare, T. (2000) 'Disabled sexuality: Toward rights and recognition', *Sexuality and Disability*, 18(3): 159–166.

Shakespeare, T. (2006) *Disability Rights and Wrongs*. Oxon: Routledge.

Shakespeare, T., Gillespie-Sells, K. and Davies, D. (1996) *The Sexual Politics of Disability: Untold Desires*. London: Continuum International Publishing Group.

Shelley, M. (2008 [1818]) *Frankenstein*. Oxford: Oxford University Press.

Shelvin, M. (2010) 'Valuing and learning from young people', in R. Rose (ed.) *Confronting Obstacles to Inclusion: International Responses to Developing Inclusive Education*. Oxon: Routledge and Nasen.

Shildrick, M. (1997) *Leaky Bodies and Boundaries: Feminism, Postmodernism and (Bio)Ethics*. London: Routledge.

Shildrick, M. (2002) *Embodying the Monster: Encounters with the Vulnerable Self*. London: Sage Publications.

Shildrick, M. (2009) *Dangerous Discourses of Disability, Subjectivity and Sexuality*. Houndmills: Palgrave Macmillan.

Sibley, D. (1995) *Geographies of Exclusion*. London: Routledge.

Siebers, T. (2012) 'A sexual culture for disabled people', in R. McRuer and A. Mollow (eds) *Sex and Disability*. London: Duke University Press.

Silvers, A. (2009) 'No talent? Beyond the worst off! A diverse theory of justice for disability', in K. Brownlee and A. Cureton (eds) *Disability and Disadvantage*. New York: Oxford University Press.

Singal, N. (2010) 'Including "children with special needs" in the Indian education system: Negotiating a contested terrain', in R. Rose (ed.) *Confronting Obstacles to Inclusion: International Responses to Developing Inclusive Education*. Oxon: Routledge and Nasen, pp. 45–57.

Slee, R. (2010) 'Revisiting the politics of special educational needs and disability studies in education with Len Barton', *British Journal of Sociology of Education*, 31(5): 561–573.

Slee, R. (2011) *The Irregular School: Exclusion, Schooling and Inclusive Education*. Oxon: Routledge.

Slee, R. (2012) 'How do we make inclusive education happen when exclusion is a political predisposition?', *International Journal of Inclusive Education*, DOI: 10.1080/13603116.2011.602534.

Smart, C. (2007) *Personal Life*. Cambridge: Polity Press.

Smart, C. and Neale, B. (1999) *Family Fragments?* Cambridge: Polity Press.

Smith, B. and Sparkes, A. C. (2005) 'Men, sport, spinal cord injury, and narratives of hope', *Social Science & Medicine*, 61: 1095–1105.

Smyth, J., Down, B. and McInerney, P. (2010) *Hanging in with the Kids in Tough Times: Engagement in Contexts of Educational Disadvantage in the Relational School*. New York: Peter Lang Publishing.

Sontag, S. (1979) *On Photography*. London: Penguin Books.

Sontag, S. (2003) *Regarding the Pain of Others*. London: Penguin Books.

Sparkes, A. C. (1994) 'Life histories and the issue of voice: Reflections on an emerging relationship', *Qualitative Studies in Education*, 7(2): 165–183.

Sparkes, A. C. (2002) 'Autoethnography: Self-indulgence or something more?' in A. Bochner and C. Ellis (eds) *Ethnographically Speaking: Autoethnography, Literature, and Aesthetics.* New York: Altamira Press.

Spencer, L. and Pahl, R. (2006) *Rethinking Friendship: Hidden Solidarities Today.* Woodstock: Princeton University Press.

Standing, E. M. (1998) *Maria Montessori: Her Life and Work.* New York: Plume Publishing.

Stanley, L. (1992) *The Auto/biographical I.* Manchester: Manchester University Press.

Stanley, L. (1993) 'On auto/biography in sociology', *Sociology*, 27(1): 41–52.

Stark, C. (2010) 'Respecting human dignity: Contract versus capabilities', in E. F. Kittay and L. Carlson (eds) *Cognitive Disability and its Challenge to Moral Philosophy.* West Sussex: Wiley-Blackwell, pp. 111–126.

Stienstra, D. and Ashcroft, T. (2010) 'Voyaging on the seas of spirit: An ongoing journey towards understanding disability and humanity', *Disability and Society*, 25(2): 191–203.

Sundaram, V. and Wilde, A. (2012) 'Investigating the value of vignettes in researching disabled students' view of social equality and inclusion in school', in Y. Taylor (ed.) *Educational Diversity: The Subject of Difference and Different Subjects.* Houndmills: Palgrave Macmillan.

Swain, J., French, S., Barnes, C. and Thomas, C. (2004) *Disabling Barriers – Enabling Environments.* London: Sage Publications.

Swift, J. (1967 [1726]) *Gulliver's Travels.* London: Penguin.

Terzi, L. (2007) 'Capability and educational equality: The just distribution of resources to students with disabilities and special educational needs', *Journal of Philosophy of Education*, 41(4): 757–773.

Terzi, L. (2009) 'Vagaries of the natural lottery? Human diversity, disability, and justice: a capability perspective', in K. Brownlee and A. Cureton (eds) *Disability and Disadvantage.* New York: Oxford University Press, pp. 86–109.

Tester, K. (2001) *Compassion, Morality and the Media.* Buckingham: Open University Press.

Theodosius, C. (2008) *Emotional Labour in Health Care: The Unmanaged Heart of Nursing.* London: Routledge.

Thomas, C. (1999) *Female Forms: Experiencing and Understanding Disability.* Buckingham: Open University Press.

Thomas, C. (2007) *Sociologies of Disability and Illness: Contested Ideas in Disability Studies and Medical Sociology.* Basingstoke: Palgrave Macmillan.

Thomas, P. (2011) '"Mate crime": Ridicule, hostility and targeted attacks against disabled people', *Disability and Society*, 26(1) 107–111.

Thomas, P. (2013) 'Hate crime or mate crime? Disablist hostility, contempt and ridicule', in A. Roulstone and H. Mason-Bish (eds) *Disability, Hate Crime and Violence.* Oxon: Routledge.

Tissot, C. (2011) 'Working together? Parent and local authority views on the process of obtaining appropriate educational provision for children with autism spectrum disorders', *Educational Research*, 53(1): 1–15.

Tomlinson, S. (2013) *Ignorant Yobs? Low Attainers in a Global Knowledge Economy.* Oxon: Routledge.

Topping, K. and Maloney, S. (2005) (eds) *The Routledge Falmer Reader in Inclusive Education.* London: Routledge.

Tronto, J. (1989) 'Women and caring: What can feminists learn about morality from caring?', in A. M. Jaggar and S. Bordo (eds) *Gender/Body/Knowledge: Feminist Reconstructions of Being and Knowing.* New Brunswick and London: Rutgers University Press.

Tronto, J. (1993a) *Moral Boundaries: A Political Argument for an Ethic of Care.* London: Routledge.

Tronto, J. (1993b) 'Beyond gender difference to a theory of care', in M. J. Larrabee (ed.) *An Ethic of Care: Feminist and Interdisciplinary Perspectives.* London: Routledge.

Tronto, J. (2011) 'A feminist democractic ethics of care and global care workers', in R. Mahon and F. Robinson (eds) *Feminist Ethics and Social Policy: Towards a New Global Political Economy of Care.* Canada: University of British Columbia Press.

Tronto, J. and Fisher, B. (1990) 'Towards a feminist theory of caring', in K. Abel and M. Nelson (eds) *Circles of Care.* New York: SUNY Press.

Turner, G. and Crane, E. (in press) 'Sexually silenced no more: adults with intellectual disabilities speak about pleasure', *Sexualities.*

Turton, J. (2007) *Child Abuse, Gender and Society.* London: Routledge.

UNESCO (2011) *UNESCO and Education: Everyone has the Right to Education.* France: United Nations Educational, Scientific and Cultural Organisation.

Utting, R. (2015) 'Disability Cuts: Tory brutality in full swing', *The People's Assembly.* Available from: http://www.thepeoplesassembly.org.uk/disability_cuts_tory_bruta lity_in_full_swing (accessed 5 August 2015).

Vanhoozer, K. (1990) *Biblical Narrative in the Philosophy of Paul Ricoeur: A Study in Hermeneutics and Theology.* Cambridge: Cambridge University Press.

Ve, H. (1989) 'The male gender roles and responsibility for children', in K. Boh, M. Bak, C. Clason, M. Pankratova, J. Qvortrup, B. Giovanni and K. Waerness (eds) *Changing Patterns of European Family Life: A Comparative Analysis of 14 European Countries.* London and New York: Routledge.

Vincent, C. (2000) *Including Parents? Education, Citizenship and Parental Agency.* Buckingham: Open University Press.

Vorhaus, J. (2016) *Giving Voice to Profound Disability: Dignity, Dependent and Human Capabilities.* London: Routledge.

Walker, P. (2009) 'Incident diary reveals ordeal of mother who killed herself and daughter', *The Guardian.* 24 September. Available at: http://www.theguardian.com/ uk/2009/sep/24/fiona-pilkington-incident-diary (accessed 5 August 2015).

Walker, P. and Quinn, B. (2012) 'UKIP suspends election candidate after "abhorrent" abortion remark', *The Guardian.* Available from: http://www.theguardian.com/politics/ 2012/dec/18/ukip-candidate-abortion-for-downs-syndrome (accessed 5 August 2015).

Walker, M. and Unterhalter, E. (2007) (eds) *Amartya Sen's Capability Approach and Social Justice in Education.* Houndmills: Palgrave Macmillan.

Watkins, A. and Meijer, C. (2010) 'The development of inclusive teaching and learning: A European perspective?', in R. Rose (ed.) *Confronting Obstacles to Inclusion: International Responses to Developing Inclusive Education.* Oxon: Routledge and Nasen.

Wearmouth, J. (ed.) (2001) *Special Educational Provision in the Context of Inclusion.* London: David Fulton.

Wilkinson, I. (2005) *Suffering: A Sociological Introduction.* Cambridge: Polity Press.

Withnall, A. (2014) 'Lord Freud disabled wage comments: "Those words will haunt him", say Tory MPs as peer faces calls to resign', *The Independent.* Available from:

http://www.independent.co.uk/news/uk/politics/lord-freud-disabled-wage-comments-those-words-will-haunt-him-say-tory-mps-as-peer-faces-calls-to-resign-9796525.html (accessed 5 August 2015).

Woodthorpe, K. (2011) 'Researching death: Methodological reflections on the management of critical distance', *International Journal of Social Research Methodology*, 14(2): 99–109.

Wolff, J. (2002) *Why Read Marx Today*. New York: Oxford University Press.

Wolff, J. (2009) 'Disability among equals', in K. Brownlee and A. Cureton (eds) *Disability and Disadvantage*. New York: Oxford University Press, pp. 112–136.

Wolff, J. and De-Shalit, A. (2007) *Disadvantage*. Oxford: Oxford University Press.

Wright Mills, C. (1959) *The Sociological Imagination*. New York: Oxford University Press.

Yar, M. and Rafter, N. (2013) 'Justice for the disabled: Crime films on punishment and the human rights of people with learning disabilities', in A. Wagner and R. K. Sherwin (eds) *Law, Culture and Visual Studies*. New York: Springer.

Young, I. M. (1990 [2011]) *Justice and the Politics of Difference*. Oxfordshire: Princetown University Press.

Young, I. M. (2000) *Inclusion and Democracy*. New York: Oxford University Press.

Young, J. (1999) *The Exclusive Society*. London: Sage.

Young, J. (2007) *The Vertigo of Late Modernity*. London: Sage.

Index

Ahmed, S. 19
alienation: in the act of production 29–30; from human to human 30; Marx's theory of 28–31; from object of production 29; from species being 30
Allan, J. 73–80, 82
animal rights 47
Arendt, H. 2–3

Baker, J. 84, 95
beings-in-relation 39
Benjamin, S. 82
Berger, J. 10, 16–17
Berube, M. 48–9
bodies: disgust and fears of contamination 9–10, 17; and hegemony of normalcy 4–5, 77; social aversion to difficult bodies 132
Boyne, John (*The Boy in the Striped Pyjamas*) 9
Breaking Bad 12–13, 139

capabilities approach: application to education 47, 81–2; basic capabilities 45; combined capabilities 45; concept overview 40–5; critiques of 48–9; human rights approach and 40–1; internal capabilities 45–6; relationality and 48; social justice approach and 42–3, 47–8; ten central capabilities 42–3, 81–2
capitalism 28–31
Carabine, J. 77, 131
care ethics model of disability: care ethics and the law 53–5; caring relations as pluralistic 41, 56, 82; caring relations foundation of 52–3; the caring spheres 137–8; for education 84–6; and employment 32; interdependence and

relationality 44–5, 51; and markers of care 54–5; overview of 31–2, 34, 41–2; the psycho-social within 138–40; relationships and institutions interplay 49–50
caring: boundaries for professional workers 116–17, 122–6; care-giver/care-receiver relationship 36, 52; caring for vs. caring about distinction 30, 36–7, 54, 94–5, 104, 110; economic issues and 22–3; natural vs. ethical caring 36, 94, 110; as pluralistic practice 41, 56, 82; relationship with ethic of justice 37–8
Carlson, L. 18–19
Carrabine, E. 11, 14, 133
citizenship: exclusion of the intellectually disabled from 2, 47–8, 81; value of care in relation to 37
community: citizenship and feminist care ethic 37; human interactions and 3, 30; human relationships and production 28
consumerism 69–70
contractarianism 45
Crane, E. 114
Cremin, C. 11

Davis, L. J. 4
dehumanisation: dysfunctional labelling 86–7; and employment opportunities 32; images in the media 15–17; of the intellectually disabled 2, 15, 18–19, 48; and intimate relationships 117; Marx's theory of alienation and 29–30; and the need for social interaction 3; and normalisation processes 77, 134; and opportunities for friendships 124–5
Derek 127–8

Made in the USA
Middletown, DE
26 August 2020